THE
EVERYTHING®

ORGASM BOOK

Dear Reader,

What a gift for me to be able to share this information
with you! I feel blessed to have this opportunity to write
so much about a subject I feel so strongly about. I hope
to make some difference in the lives of my readers who
are searching for more information on a topic so rarely
talked about at length in any real or informative way.

The path I have followed as a clinical sexologist has
taken me to many interesting places and presented many
new challenges. I have embraced this one fully with
excitement and gusto, thinking of the lives I could touch
and the sexualities I could help liberate and expand into
whole new territories of discovery—and ultimately pleasure.

For me, the orgasmic experience is one of total
release and surrender, and it has a life of its own. It too
yearns for growth and expansion. It wants to find new
heights and greater depths. This book is intended to support that growth and expansion so that your orgasmic
experience can keep improving. May you find yourself in
ever-increasing orgasmic bliss!

Amy Cooper, PhD

Welcome to the EVERYTHING Series!

These handy, accessible books give you all you need to tackle a difficult project, gain a new hobby, or even brush up on something you learned back in school but have since forgotten. You can choose to read from cover to cover or just pick out information from our four useful boxes.

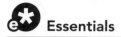 **Alerts**

Urgent warnings

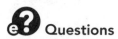 **Facts**

Important snippets of information

 Essentials

Quick handy tips

 Questions

Answers to common questions

When you're done reading, you can finally
say you know **EVERYTHING**®!

PUBLISHER Karen Cooper

DIRECTOR OF ACQUISITIONS AND INNOVATION Paula Munier

MANAGING EDITOR, EVERYTHING® SERIES Lisa Laing

COPY CHIEF Casey Ebert

ACQUISITIONS EDITOR Katrina Schroeder

ASSOCIATE DEVELOPMENT EDITOR Elizabeth Kassab

SENIOR DEVELOPMENT EDITOR Brett Palana-Shanahan

EDITORIAL ASSISTANT Hillary Thompson

EVERYTHING® SERIES COVER DESIGNER Erin Alexander

LAYOUT DESIGNERS Colleen Cunningham, Elisabeth Lariviere, Ashley Vierra, Denise Wallace

Visit the entire Everything® series at *www.everything.com*

THE
EVERYTHING®
ORGASM BOOK

The all-you-need guide to the most satisfying sex you'll ever have

Amy Cooper, PhD

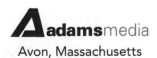
Adamsmedia
Avon, Massachusetts

To seekers of greater pleasure and bliss—there is more!

An Everything® Series Book.
Everything® and everything.com® are registered trademarks of F+W Media, Inc.

Published by Adams Media, a division of F+W Media, Inc.
57 Littlefield Street, Avon, MA 02322 U.S.A.
www.adamsmedia.com

ISBN 10: 1-60550-992-2
ISBN 13: 978-1-60550-992-1

Printed in the United States of America.

J I H G F E D C B A

Library of Congress Cataloging-in-Publication Data
is available from the publisher.

This publication is designed to provide accurate and authoritative information with regard to the subject matter covered. It is sold with the understanding that the publisher is not engaged in rendering legal, accounting, or other professional advice. If legal advice or other expert assistance is required, the services of a competent professional person should be sought.
—From a *Declaration of Principles* jointly adopted by a Committee of the American Bar Association and a Committee of Publishers and Associations

Many of the designations used by manufacturers and sellers to distinguish their products are claimed as trademarks. Where those designations appear in this book and Adams Media was aware of a trademark claim, the designations have been printed with initial capital letters.

Illustrations by Eric Andrews

*This book is available at quantity discounts for bulk purchases.
For information, please call 1-800-289-0963.*

All the examples and dialogues used in this book are fictional, and have been created by the author to illustrate particular situations.

Acknowledgments

I would like to thank my beloved family, friends, lovers, and community who have encouraged and supported me through this entire book writing process. A huge thank you to my amazing partner, Tim Hartnett, for all of the faith, support, and guidance you have offered me throughout the years, not to mention the endless hours of editing you have put into this book. A special thank you to my dear friend, Andrew Davis, for your encouragement and all of your help with the orgasm survey; and to my beloved friends, Monica Woelfel and Rebecca McCubbin, for help with editing and finishing touches. Thank you to my dear friend, Carmen Alvarez, whose support and love for me holds me up and means more to me than she may really know. Thank you to Katrina Schroeder at Adams Media for finding me and for your steady encouragement and support. And tremendous thanks to all of the other pioneers and scholars in the field of sexuality, past and present, whose courage and insight shed much needed light onto a topic that has been kept in the dark for too long.

Top 10 Keys to Improving
Your Experience of Orgasm

1. Rid yourself of any sexual shame or inhibitions.

2. Work to improve your overall health and fitness.

3. Practice relaxation and deep breathing.

4. Maintain strong but relaxed pelvic floor muscles.

5. Self-pleasure regularly.

6. Become more aware of all of your senses.

7. Explore all of your body's potential erogenous zones.

8. Practice building more sexual arousal and holding more sexual charge.

9. Be open to exploring a variety of sexual behaviors.

10. Improve your communication skills in regard to sex.

Contents

Introduction

The purpose of this book is to shed some light onto the taboo subject of sex. It was written with the intent to open minds and educate readers about arousal and orgasms. It offers to help alleviate the many fears and stigmas associated with sex. The ultimate goal is to improve the experience of sex for those who are ready. The following chapters will open your eyes to many of the false beliefs pertaining to sex and orgasm that have been a source of painful confusion to many people. It will educate you about what orgasms are and are not, how they come to be, how to make them happen, and how to make them better. It will also provide you with a greater vocabulary for talking about your experiences. The more you understand about sex and the orgasmic experience, the less you will fear it, and the more likely you will enjoy your own sexuality and grant others the freedom to enjoy theirs.

The primary focus of this book is on enriching your experience of orgasm, but it is in no way a definitive guide to all possible experiences with orgasm—that would be an impossible task. The orgasmic experience is as varied and subjective as the imagination will allow. This book does, however, delve into all of the main categories of experience with orgasm, including anatomy and physiology of orgasm, body-mind preparation, relationship and communication skills, sexual behaviors, and unique challenges. Studying and learning more in these realms can help you find your way to greater and greater arousal and orgasmic pleasure.

The information in this book will provide you with many useful tools as you explore your erotic self and seek more enjoyable orgasmic experiences. It is up to you, however, to create the time and space for your own erotic exploration. As you read, consider how you might make this more of a priority in your life. Taking time out for pleasure is perhaps the most challenging hurdle to get over. To experience more enjoyable and powerful orgasms, it is crucial to give your body the time it needs to relax into sex and build arousal. This is your journey, your unfolding into bliss, and you are the only one who can make that happen for yourself.

The time for closer examination and exploration of your sexuality is ripe. More and more brave souls are pioneering their way to greater erotic and orgasmic pleasure and sharing their discoveries, paving the way for others to do the same. There is more dialogue about sex and orgasm. The fields of clinical sexology, sex coaching, and sex therapy are growing. And there are many books, magazines, websites, and informative programs and videos available to assist you in your explorations. There is considerable momentum for tearing down the dilapidated old walls of sexual shame and ignorance and planting beautiful gardens of sexual satisfaction and enjoyment in their place. Explore the ever-expanding fields of possibility and potential for more exquisite erotic and orgasmic experiences; they are your birthright. You deserve all the pleasure you can receive!

CHAPTER 1

The Mystique of Orgasm

O rgasm is one of the most powerful and pleasurable natural experiences life offers. It is an experience that is highly sought after and celebrated, but it is also feared and repressed. The subjective experience of orgasm is different for everyone, making it something of an enigma. Many cultures throughout history have tried to define it, contain it, or liberate it. But after several thousand years of attention to the subject, there is still much to understand about its significance and its tremendous potential for pleasure.

Describing Orgasm

There are lots of ways to describe orgasms. You can reference them by what part of your body was stimulated to produce them. For example, a woman may say she had a vaginal or a clitoral orgasm as a result of vaginal or clitoral stimulation. Or you can talk about an orgasm by describing the sensations it produced, such as a warm tingling sensation, a shock wave, or a massive explosion. You might describe how an orgasm progresses in your body, such as a sequence of sensations that ripples from your genitals to your fingers and toes. Or you might describe the effect the orgasm had on your connection to your partner, such as a feeling of merging or of magnetizing with each other. Finally, your orgasm may be described in relation to a more spiritual meaning that you have given it, such as a releasing into oneness with God or the whole universe.

The following descriptions came from a survey on orgasms in response to a question asking people to describe a particularly enjoyable experience of orgasm. You can see the great variety in the responses.

I had a very deep vaginal orgasm, and it felt like loads of energy were being released through my entire body.

It was then that I felt the most stirring, fluttering, warm feeling coming through me . . . it started in my belly, came out my pussy, and just kept going and going and going. . . . There was no real ending, just a leveling off.

I felt the pleasure move completely through my body, slowly from my feet to my head, moving out through my head. I also had the sensation of strong ejaculation, as if I were a man, and that felt very powerful and strong. I felt elation and bliss progress within me, until my entire body was engaged and fully open to myself and my partner. Afterwards I cried in joy.

At that point, instead of the arousal curve dropping off, it skyrocketed, and the resulting subjective orgasm was so amazing, all encompassing, and subjectively long, that I passed out for just a moment.

. . . when I came it was like an electric shock—my eyes flew open and my body jerked wildly.

Waves upon waves. White energy bliss bubble. Breathing energy in and out. Closing an energy circle through lingam going in and coming out through her glistening eyes. Still shivering uncontrollably a few times.

I felt my skin get warm with a rush of excitement throughout my whole body moving upwards. Warm fluid released from what felt like the walls of my yoni and my cervix. I felt my connection to the universe in that moment of warmth and pleasure. It was so easeful and I was pleasantly surprised by the ease of this deep connection and pleasure. So much joy flooded our space together as we realized the level of connection we were creating.

There is no right or wrong way to describe orgasms. And there is no single description that will work for every orgasm. There is a certain degree of subjectivity with each individual orgasm that can only truly be described in a narrative form, and chances are even that touches lightly on the actual experience of orgasm.

The Meaning of Orgasm

What does orgasm mean to you? Why do you have orgasms, or try to? Is it important if you do or don't? Understanding the meaning of orgasm for you can help you focus on what you are really after in the experience. Are you doing it for pleasure, for procreation, for love? Just like descriptions of orgasm, the meanings people find in orgasm vary widely. We are influenced by both our culture and by our personal experiences. And we each end up with our own take on this mysterious phenomenon.

 Fact

La petit mort is a French expression often used to refer to orgasm. It literally means *the small death*. The meaning that this infers is that essentially a part of the self dies or is released in the experience of orgasm. And indeed many people find this to be true.

One response to the survey said, "It is the 'small death' that reveals the essence of aliveness. Alone, in masturbation, it can be everything from simply a means to an end (relaxation, sleep, focus) to a deep affirmation of my love for myself. Shared, it creates and strengthens the bond with my partner. There is something in it of ritual, transformation, or journey. A place outside of all regular places where I meet my lover stripped bare of everything but my most simple self."

This response touches on a number of common themes. Many of the other responses spoke to the following aspects of meaning:

- Emotional, energetic, and sexual release. Most people think of orgasms as providing some sort of emotional, energetic or sexual release. It is a letting go of pent-up energy, a flowing forth, a spilling over.
- Relaxation tool and sleep aid. Many people find that orgasms are an excellent tool for stress reduction and seek them out as a way to relax or fall asleep.
- Symbol of love, intimacy, and connection. Orgasms can also be a symbol for the profound expression of love and connection you have with a lover.
- Sexual freedom. For some, having orgasms symbolizes their sexual freedom. They are free to follow their sexual urges all the way to orgasmic bliss or release.
- Openness to deep pleasure and intensity. For some, the orgasmic experience demonstrates the ability to surrender to profound pleasure. It is a symbol of willingness to embrace the intensity of sensation and, on some level, life itself.
- Culmination of excitement and desire. Orgasms can also signify the termination of excitement and desire. Some embrace this as a wonderful state, while others may feel sad that all of the passion and the intense connection has come to an end.

- Spiritual doorway to an expanded self. For some, orgasms hold a spiritual significance and are a portal to their more expanded selves. They are a way to experience a connection to all that exists.

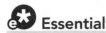 **Essential**

Whatever meaning you give to the orgasmic experience can be different depending on the kind of sexual behavior, the nature of a particular relationship, or the type or quality of the orgasm itself. It can also change through the course of your life. Your sexuality is variable and malleable.

Here are some more examples of the different meanings survey respondents give to orgasm:

"It can be an experience of pure animal consciousness, of wanting and taking and submitting and releasing. Losing myself in touch and blood and bone."

"Having orgasms means I am open to pleasure, intensity and eroticism, that I trust my body's wisdom, and that I acknowledge my right to enjoy myself as much as I am capable of."

"To be honest, it can be a disappointment. As wonderful as it feels, it rings the closing bell on making love (at least for a while). I often come out of the bliss state and plunge into self-doubt and recrimination."

"It all depends on the context. If I'm by myself (which is most often), then it's a goal. I pleasure myself with the goal of having an orgasm. The orgasm itself can fill many needs—relaxation, stress relief, preparation for sleep, and even a drug. It also has a spiritual/energetic function as in Tantric sex. If I'm with a partner in a love relationship, then orgasm for me

is more of an ornament—a culmination of all the affection, connection, and energetic play that comes before it. Whether orgasm comes and how soon (or how long it lasts) is secondary. This helps me be more open to the experience in all its unique aspects, which opens up my romantic, sexual, and orgasmic capabilities."

"They show me how it is possible to go beyond myself and dissipate in the all that is. Somehow, they seem like a reward for sharing myself, either with someone else or with the universe in a certain way. When I have them on my own, I'm very intentional about it."

"For me, it is the ultimate enjoyment of life in this body. It can take on forms of worship and symbolize uniting with the one at that moment of bliss. It can be an expression for love of the other, or love of yourself. Sometimes it is just experiencing pleasure in this physical realm."

The meanings that people give to their orgasms are as unique and varied as the people themselves. They are windows into their souls and show the diversity within each person and among different people. It is important to allow for these kinds of personal narratives when discussing sex, for they get to the heart of the matter and display what is really essential about orgasm for many people.

Myths about Orgasm

In order to understand what orgasms are and how you can best enjoy them, it is useful to understand what they are not. Chances are you have been exposed to all kinds of myths about sex and orgasm since you were a child. These myths have caused a lot of pain and confusion for some people.

When asked about myths pertaining to orgasm, one survey respondent shared one of the most common misperceptions about sex: "I was told as a child not to touch my genitals, that they were dirty. I didn't stop touching myself, but I always felt ashamed about it and I was afraid of getting caught. The myths that my genitals were dirty and that masturbation was shameful have taken me awhile to overcome."

Common Myths

Ridding yourself of any limiting or false beliefs or attitudes about orgasms is truly the first step on your path to enriched orgasmic experiences. If a belief is engrained or embedded into your psyche, it may take some time and experience to undo it, but it is a worthwhile journey. Here are some more common myths that may be limiting your enjoyment of orgasm in some way.

Vaginal intercourse or penetration is the only real route to orgasm.

One survey respondent noted, "I used to be really upset when I couldn't make my partner reach orgasm with just vaginal intercourse. I thought that if my penis was in and doing the right thing that I should make her orgasm and if I didn't I failed. I thought that if I had to use my hands to stimulate the clitoris while I was having sex that I was cheating or something. I have long lost this notion and currently use my hands all the time, no matter where my penis is."

The truth is that there are very clearly many routes to orgasm. Men and women both can enjoy orgasms by engaging in numerous kinds of sexual behavior. There is no proven better or more appropriate way to achieve orgasm.

"I thought that vaginal penetration was the ticket to orgasm, but this has turned out to be a myth," one survey respondent said. "I do not feel like this had any effect my experience of orgasm because I still orgasm without penetration. I thought phalluses had to be involved (silicone or otherwise), but it turns out I like hands and mouths better."

Orgasms can only last a few seconds.

There are many different kinds of orgasms and orgasmic experiences that vary in intensity and duration. Some orgasmic states and experiences can last much longer than a few seconds.

Orgasms should all be "earth shaking."

Every orgasm has the potential to be meaningful and pleasurable, regardless of its intensity. Some are mellow, some are quiet, some are short, some are profound, some are loud, and some are long. Great or small, each one should be considered a gift.

Women can't orgasm as much as men.

It is true that women often have a more difficult time finding their way to orgasm, at least initially; however, once they do, their access to multiple orgasms is much greater than men's. In fact, women on the whole are capable of being much more orgasmic than men.

Clitoral orgasms are immature and inferior to vaginal orgasms.

There is no such thing as an immature or inferior orgasm! The quality of your orgasm is not solely a factor of what is being stimulated. In fact, the intensity of orgasm is much more a factor of how open you are to receiving pleasure in whatever form it is administered.

Orgasms are the goal of sex.

As amazing as orgasms are, there is no reason why sex has to include orgasmic release. Sex can be very pleasurable, ecstatic, and meaningful without culminating in an orgasm.

Orgasm in men is always accompanied by ejaculation.

Men are capable of having an orgasm without ejaculation. Some men learn by chance to separate orgasm and ejaculation. Others can learn with practice.

If you are a man, orgasms that include ejaculation will deplete your energy.

There are some belief systems that purport that a man's life energy is depleted when he ejaculates. Some men may find this to be true, but there are many men who ejaculate frequently who do not find that it depletes their energy in any way. In fact, some men find that it keeps them vital.

If you self-pleasure you will lose desire or interest in being with a lover.

Just because you are capable of providing yourself with orgasms does not mean you will lose interest in being with a lover. The need for intimacy and connection with another cannot be met by being alone. Also the experience of orgasm with a lover can be a very different experience than what you experience when you are by yourself.

A man is responsible for helping a woman achieve orgasm.

Some men feel like they are failures if they do not provide their female lover with an orgasm. Because women's orgasmic responses are so unique and complex, it is important that they ultimately take responsibility for their own orgasm. Your desire and willingness to learn how to help provide an orgasm should be appreciated but not expected.

You shouldn't have to use your hands to achieve or provide an orgasm.

The idea that using your hands to assist in or achieve an orgasm is somehow cheating or wrong should definitely be thrown out the window. All that matters is whatever feels good and whatever works.

Alert

Don't believe everything you hear or read, especially when it pertains to sex and orgasm. Many myths are generated and perpetuated by people with limited experience or knowledge about orgasms. Other myths spring from the culture's mores about sex and what appropriate sexual behaviors are.

If you want to liberate your sexuality, you must first free your mind from these limiting and false beliefs. Many myths survive partly due to the great discomfort people have with talking about sex in a frank and open manner. Therefore, the more you can open your mind and speak freely about your experiences, the more myths pertaining to sex and orgasm you will put to rest.

Life's Variety

Sex and orgasms have been around since the beginning of life. Nobody invented them. They have always been a part of the human experience. Cultures around the world have had their own evolving views, attitudes, and behaviors pertaining to sex and orgasm. Some of these have been openly acknowledged and written about. Others have been shrouded in secrecy or cloaked in shame.

In order to more thoroughly understand human sexual behavior, it can help to look at the sexual behaviors of other species, as well as different cultures. In doing this, you begin to see how variable and adaptable sexual behavior really is. In the bigger picture—the greater scheme—there is no such thing as normal sexual behavior. There are many paths to orgasm, many reasons for going there, many ways to describe it, and many meanings to give it. The following are a sample of life's varieties of sexual behavior.

 Fact

All female mammals have clitorises and are therefore presumably biologically capable of achieving orgasm. It is believed, however, that most female mammals do not typically experience orgasm, at least not in the way that female humans and some primates do. This belief is based primarily on the study of the facial expressions and bodily reactions of females during mating.

Our Primate Relatives

The variety of sexual practices in the animal kingdom is mind-boggling. One particularly interesting example is seen in our closest primate relatives—the bonobos. These small African apes have been studied extensively in the last few decades, partially because of their distinctive sexual behaviors. Sex among the bonobos has a variety of purposes aside from procreation; it is used to appease one another, to reconcile differences, to express affection, to reduce stress, to claim social status, and for sheer erotic excitement and pleasure. Also, sex among the bonobos occurs in nearly every imaginable partner combination, including female-to-female and male-to-male, and even mixed groups. Although it is uncertain as to whether the female bonobos actually experience orgasm like some other close primate relatives—notably chimpanzees and macaques—it is clear that they enjoy their sexual interactions and seek them out almost constantly.

Ancient Human Practices

Human history is also full of a great variety of sexual norms and practices. One example is the Ancient Babylonian women who devoted themselves to Ishtar, the goddess of love, fertility, and war. Ishtar's temple priestesses were, essentially, sacred prostitutes. Male travelers would go to Ishtar's temple to make offerings to the goddess and then be worshipped and made love to by temple priestesses. It was also a custom for all women to go to the temple of Ishtar at least once. Each woman would sit until a traveler threw a coin in her lap. Then she would go off and have sex with the stranger before returning home to get married and start a family. This was considered a rite of passage that would help with fertility. It was also believed to ward off future temptations to sleep around.

Cultural Variations

Every culture, ancient and modern, has its own views and norms on sex. The Polynesians in particular, however, have been known for their more liberated attitudes toward sex. In ancient Polynesia, sexual relations started very early in life and were very frequent and varied. There was little about sex that was considered taboo. Although this situation has changed somewhat in modern times, Polynesian attitudes pertaining to sex are still more open than those of many other cultures.

Today, the Polynesians have a reputation of being more slow and languid in their sexual encounters and lovemaking. They do not hurry toward orgasm. In fact, they are more likely to postpone it in order to enjoy all of the delightful feelings and sensations in their bodies, including the love they have for their partner. In *Slow Love: A Polynesian Pillow Book*, James N. Powell elaborates on this deliciously slow and sensual way of lovemaking.

Variations from the Norm

Even when there is a strong norm within a culture, deviations from that norm can be prevalent. Monogamy, for example, is a norm most human cultures encourage. In practice, however, many people do not confine their quest for sexual pleasure and orgasmic experiences to one person. Some people do this openly. Others keep it hidden. Such non-monogamy ranges widely, from illicit affairs to polyamorous relationships and group sex parties. Others are happy to have and keep just one lover for their entire life.

 Essential

Polyamory is the name given to the conscious practice of having more than one lover or partner at a time. People choosing to adopt a polyamorous lifestyle tend to value honesty and integrity in their relationships. It is not a fear of commitment that motivates them to have more than one lover. They simply want to love more.

The Politics of Orgasm

As powerful and wonderful as sex and orgasms can be, they are also strongly feared and often repressed. Throughout history and across cultures, there have been attempts to restrict, limit, or altogether abolish certain sexual behaviors. These restrictions have been executed in a variety of ways; sometimes through ridicule or shaming, sometimes with the threat of losing status or being excluded from the group or tribe, and sometimes with the threat of fines, imprisonment, injury, or even death. There have also been many attempts to liberate sexuality from such repressive views and attitudes.

Sex Laws

Laws pertaining to sexual behavior have been around since the beginning of civilization. The first evidence of rules pertaining to sexual behavior dates back to the beginning of the early Ancient Egyptians in the form of pictographs and pictograms. Later, written laws grew increasingly specific about adultery, sexual abuse, rape, incest, anal sex, oral sex, homosexuality, age of consent, prostitution, and bestiality. Some of these laws probably seemed quite necessary and reasonable to the majority of people. Many of them, however, seem to exist solely to control the sexual behaviors of others, even behaviors in which there are two consenting adults, and no harm is being done.

 Fact

The Hammurabi Code—the oldest written laws known to mankind—included the first written sex laws. It dates back to the eighteenth century B.C. in the ancient civilization of Babylon and includes laws pertaining to adultery, rape, and incest. It says nothing of homosexuality or prostitution; laws concerning these practices did not come until later in the history of civilization.

There are still many antiquated sex laws in the United States today. Most of them, such as laws criminalizing adultery and oral or anal sex, are rarely enforced. Because they are so rarely enforced, there is little incentive to change them. It is essential, however, to keep laws current with the culture's changing attitudes. This will, in the long run, protect those who may fall prey to the lingering repressive attitudes of those who want to control the sexual behavior of others.

Some cultures also have laws that force people to be sexual. Women are, in some places, required by law to have sex with their husbands whenever they are approached. Men may be required to have sex with their wives every so many days or every few months. While it is great to encourage sex among married couples, enforcing it is a kind of sexual repression. People need to be free to make their own choices and do what feels right, when they are ready.

Clitoridectomy

The sexual repression of women has been one of the main ways that human sexuality has been subject to control by others. The means by which female sexuality has been repressed are many, but none is so physically overt than the practice of clitoridectomy. Also referred to as *female circumcision, infibulation,* or *female genital mutilation,* clitoridectomy is a procedure performed on females primarily to prevent them from experiencing sexual desire, pleasure, or orgasm. Other peripheral reasons are to preserve chastity and virginity, to symbolize social status or belonging to the group, for hygienic motivations, for male approval, and for mystical and ritualistic purposes.

Clitoridectomy is the partial or full removal of the female's external genitals, potentially including the clitoral hood, glans, and shaft, as well as the inner labia. The procedure is usually performed on young girls before they hit puberty. There are cases, however, where it has been performed on grown women, usually before or immediately after marrying into a family that practices the tradition. Clitoridectomies are usually performed without the use of an anesthetic and are often followed by immediate complications and long-term problems in regard to both the physical and mental health of the girl or woman.

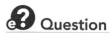 **Question**

Can women who have had a clitoridectomy still achieve orgasm?
Yes, sometimes they can. There are accounts of women who have had clitoridectomies who indeed experience vaginal orgasms through vaginal penetration alone. Also, not all of the clitoral tissue is actually removed—usually just the glans and the shaft. The clitoral bulbs remain intact and are capable of engorgement and sexual pleasure.

Clitoridectomy is a cultural practice, not a religious one. It takes place today primarily among certain groups of people in Africa, the Middle East, Indonesia, and Malaysia. Immigrants from these areas have brought the practice to other parts of the world, including the United Sates. It is believed that this practice affects more than 100 million women. The practice itself dates far back in history, since before Islam or Christianity even existed, and has been practiced by Muslims, Jews, and Christians. Only a little over 100 years ago, clitoridectomies were performed in the United States and Britain as treatment for excessive masturbation, lesbianism, hysteria, epilepsy, and melancholy. The practice of clitoridectomy is no longer accepted in Western culture, and there are numerous groups who are attempting to end this practice worldwide.

Although the clitoris is known to be a woman's main route to orgasm, it is not the sole route, and women who have had a clitoridectomy may still be physiologically capable of orgasm. However, it can make orgasm considerably more difficult. Still, where it is the cultural norm, women may accept it and even believe it is necessary. In order for this practice to change, many cultural views and attitudes pertaining to sexuality will have to shift.

The Sexual Revolution

The sexual revolution of the 1960s and 1970s helped unravel some of the negative attitudes pertaining to sex that had built up since the sexually repressive Victorian era. Although the sexual revolution didn't sprout until the 1960s, many of its seeds were planted a decade earlier. Sex researcher Alfred Kinsey published his now famous works on human sexual behavior in 1948 and 1953. His works mark the onset of the sexual revolution. Before these books, people were mostly in the dark about the sexual behaviors of others. Helped by Kinsey's extensive data, people began to see that they were not alone in their proclivities. They could relax and accept more of their own sexuality. Many taboo behaviors, such as masturbation and homosexuality, were normalized as a result of Kinsey's work.

Many other sex researchers and pioneers followed suit, helping to support the sexual revolution through books, workshops, seminars, and lectures. Notable contributions to the sexual revolution include Shere Hite's extensive reports on female sexuality, Masters and Johnson's study of the human sexual response, Helen Singer

Kaplan's and Hartman and Fithian's work in the area of sexual dysfunction, Betty Dodson and Lonnie Barbach's writing on female sexuality and orgasm, Bernie Zilbergeld's book on male sexuality, and Alex Comfort's guide to lovemaking. All of these researchers and pioneers have helped in the understanding, acceptance, and improvement of human sexual behavior and paved the way for continued study, research, dialogue, and exploration.

Your Orgasm

Somewhere in the great range of ways people experience sex and orgasm lies your personal experience. Perhaps you have never had an orgasm. Or maybe you want your orgasms to be easier to attain, or more satisfying. You might be curious about how other people experience orgasm. Or maybe you want to help your lover get more enjoyment from his orgasms. Whatever your interest, keep in mind the following two principles.

1. There is no right or wrong way for consenting adults to be sexual. Whatever works for you to really enjoy the gift of sexuality is most important. There is a great range of variety in other people's sexual behaviors, but none of this need dictate what is true for you. You are the ultimate authority on your own sexuality.

2. An open mind can help you find even more satisfaction with sex. There is nothing that you should do. But if you are open to exploring new sexual possibilities, you may bring yourself more and more joy and fulfillment through sex. Casting off the shackles of shame that inhibit you and allowing yourself to wholeheartedly feast on all that sex has to offer can be the most rewarding growth you will ever experience. Be free.

CHAPTER 2

Tuning Your Instrument

Think of your body as a musical instrument. Visualize a cello, a guitar, or any type of instrument you particularly love to hear. If your body actually were this instrument, then satisfying sex is perhaps the most sensuous music this instrument can play. In this analogy, orgasm could be considered the dramatic climax of that sweet music. Maybe that explains the old pickup line, "We could make beautiful music together."

The Body-Mind Instrument

Any instrument can make a sound, but in order for it to make beautiful music, it needs to be well tuned. Having orgasms (and having great orgasms, in particular) requires some basic groundwork, some tuning of your body-mind instrument. There are many things you can do to keep your instrument in good condition. Perhaps you have tuned some strings but not others. This chapter is your opportunity to consider the different ways to care for your instrument so that you can better enjoy playing its most sultry tunes.

The instrument you play when you have sex is part body and part mind. Throughout history, philosophers have attempted to differentiate the mind from the body. The more science learns about human anatomy and function, however, the more it becomes clear that the two are in fact not separate. The mind is not just the brain and the thoughts inside your head. It is the entire nervous system that spreads throughout your body. It takes in sensory information from both the environment outside of your body—through the skin, eyes, nose, mouth, and ears—and from the sensations inside your body.

Your thoughts, attitudes, fantasies, and states of mind exert a strong influence on your emotions and your responses to sexual touch. Likewise, the condition of your body affects how you view yourself, what it judges about sex, and what it is open to enjoying. Consider the unfortunate scenario of a man desiring sex but anxious about whether he will be able to maintain an erection. Is his mind affecting his penis or is his penis affecting his mind? The answer is probably both, for in sex, the body and mind function as a single unit. The well-tuned body-mind is one in which the body supports the mind and the mind supports the body.

 Fact

In recent years, the fields of neuroscience and cognitive psychology have argued that the separation of mind and body, or Cartesian Dualism, is no longer a viable model of reality. In other words, the notion that a person's intelligence, or faculty of the mind, has no connection to the physical body has been discredited.

Sex-Positive and Shame-Free

Let's look first at your overall attitude about sex and your own sexuality. Society gives very contradictory messages about sex. Some people claim that sex is inherently shameful, is only excusable for procreation, and should never be used for pleasure. On the other end of the spectrum are those who claim that unbridled sexual freedom is the only way to psychological and societal health. Most people maintain views somewhere between these extremes. Sexologists have reached a general consensus that healthy sexual functioning is aided by what they call a *sex-positive perspective*. The term essentially refers to a position that affirms the following beliefs:

- Sexual exploration and expression between two consenting adults is a basic human right, regardless of the sexual behaviors being engaged in.
- Acceptance of human sexuality can have a positive effect on both individuals and society in general.
- People have the right to straightforward and factual information about sexual health.
- It is inappropriate to judge, inhibit, or restrict other adults' consensual choices on how to have sex, who to have sex with, or how one defines their sexual identity or orientation.
- Sexual education should focus not only on disease prevention and prevention of sexual assault or unwanted pregnancy, but also on the positive aspects of sexuality, such as sexual pleasure.
- Sexuality is largely a social construct and there are few if any essential truths about sex.

If you tend to agree with all of these statements, then congratulations! You can consider your attitudes to be sex-positive. If you are challenged by any of these statements, it doesn't necessarily mean you are sex-negative, but you may want to take a closer look at some of your underlying beliefs and/or fears about sexuality. This exploration can help to resolve any difficulty or discomfort you have with sex or in experiencing orgasm.

Being fully sex-positive in both attitude and practice may not be as easy as you think. While you may not be aware of any sex-negative beliefs, you must consider more than your rational, conscious mind. Consciously, you may be very accepting and allowing of any sexual behavior between two consenting adults. But there is another level—the level of the unconscious mind. Most people are still unconsciously under the influence of old beliefs about right and wrong behavior. If your own sexual exploration is inhibited based on some negative gut reaction to a particular sexual behavior that you have never tried, then you are quite possibly suffering from the fallout of a society-imposed sexually repressed mindset. In other words, you may have some shame around sex.

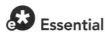 **Essential**

> Your state of mind and your attitudes pertaining to sex are integral to your enjoyment of orgasmic pleasure. Being sex-positive contributes not only to society's ease and comfort with sexual matters, but it makes a significant difference to your own inner landscape. Saying *yes* to sexuality in your mind translates to *yes* to orgasms in your body.

Shame is a painful experience caused by judgments about who you are or what you feel. These judgments originate from the attitudes of other people. You are not born believing that your body is shameful. But as a child, you are exposed to many sex-negative messages, such as "never be seen naked," "never touch yourself there," and "sex is nasty and dirty." Even if you do not believe them, these judgments can become internalized over time. Consequently, most people end up feeling bad about some aspect of their sexuality.

The feeling of shame is one of distress and humiliation. The judgments you have internalized may lead you to believe that it is inappropriate to have sexual feelings or seek sexual gratification. Simply being a part of this culture is enough to infuse you with a great deal of negativity pertaining to sexuality. This sexual shame usually resides deep in your psyche, controlling your sexual behaviors and attitudes from its stronghold inside of you. It can put a big damper on your ability to enjoy any erotic feelings. You may still have sexual feelings, but the guilt you feel about having them will take its toll on your psyche and your ability to enjoy sex and have pleasurable orgasms.

 Alert

> Sexual shame has many disguises. It masquerades as righteousness and propriety. Don't be fooled! Watch out for feelings of moral superiority, criticism, and judgment in regard to other people's sexual behaviors. They are sure signs of sexual shame lurking in your unconscious mind.

Fortunately, it is possible for you to become shame-free and relieve yourself of the psychic chains of a culturally repressed sexuality. To do so, however, requires sincere self-reflection and a willingness to open your mind, even if it is uncomfortable. Clearing out unconscious shame takes awareness, compassion, and courage. But it can be fun too. Exploring the edges of your comfort zone will both help you become shame-free and open the doors to some wonderful new sexual experiences. To begin, consider the following questions pertaining to your attitudes about sex:

- Do you feel 100 percent okay about seeking sexual pleasure with yourself and another?
- Are you willing to try new sexual behaviors?
- Do you find certain sexual behaviors inherently distasteful?
- Do you judge others for engaging in particular sexual behaviors?
- Can you talk about sex openly with your lover, spouse, friends, and/or family?

Self Reflect

The first step in moving toward a sex-positive and shame-free attitude is self-reflection. Self-reflection refers to the process of looking inward and fostering a willingness to learn more about your more subtle thoughts, beliefs, and feelings. Self-reflection is a process that helps people learn more about themselves. This is the foundation of personal growth. Self-reflecting on your attitudes and beliefs about sex will help you identify and clear shame, resulting in a greater ability to enjoy sex and orgasm to your fullest potential.

Charting your inner landscape can be challenging and scary at times. There are sometimes dark and uncomfortable feelings lurking inside. You may be tempted to avoid all of that unknown territory inside of you, because it is just too overwhelming. This is a natural response to fear. If this process is truly overwhelming, consider consulting with a clinical sexologist or a therapist. But make sure the therapist you choose has sex-positive attitudes herself. You can assess this by asking some direct questions about sex and seeing how comfortable the therapist is in response. Also note how accepted you feel about your sexuality.

> **EXERCISE:** Journal entry. Consider who and what shaped your sexual attitudes. Are any of these attitudes a source of shame? Ask yourself what could possibly be wrong with safely experiencing sexual pleasure. Open a dialogue between the part of you that wants acceptance of your sexuality and the part of you that still feels shame and limits your sexual exploration.

Expand Your Mind

The second step in becoming truly sex-positive and shame-free is to challenge any limiting beliefs you may have about sex. Some of these limitations will arise through your self-reflection on the topic. You may be someone who is not daunted by the journey inward and the study of your own perceptions. But are you open to the variety of sexual possibilities that you have not yet experienced? Expanding your mind means doing a little research outside your comfort zone.

Perhaps you are reluctant or scared to look outside of yourself for answers or new information. You may lack trust in the knowledge and experience of others. Or perhaps your ego gets in the way of allowing another person to be the expert or simply have something of value to offer you. If any of these ideas are true for you, then ask yourself why you would limit yourself to information coming only from within. What is keeping you from allowing other explorers of sexual pleasure from influencing you in some way?

Expanding your mind is easier today than ever before, although not all neighborhoods and communities are places where this can happen so readily. There are, however, a plethora of books, videos, websites, radio talk shows, and even television shows available to support your erotic exploration. There are also workshops that are designed specifically for enriching your sex life. Stores have knowledgeable staff that cater to your erotic needs. They sell books, toys, lube, props, and costumes, and even offer educational classes and workshops on sexuality. There is no need to stay stuck in a rut with your sexuality when there are so many resources available to you.

> **EXERCISE:** Consider some sexual activity or behavior that you have never tried and are perhaps a bit wary of—for example, anal sex. Do some research on the topic. Get a book or video and learn something about it and then decide whether or not to give it a try.

Talk to Others

The third step is to find people you know who are open to discussing sexuality in a new and enlightened way. Talking to a lover or to friends about your attitudes and views about sex can help you both clarify how you feel and possibly give you new perspectives that you would not otherwise have accessed. Hearing people you know describe their sexuality can help give you courage to articulate your own feelings and desires.

If you don't know of anyone to do this with, consider using the Internet to help you connect with others who are also exploring new horizons in the realm of sexual attitudes and behaviors. There are also a growing number of sex therapists and clinical sexologists who are able to assist your growth process. Ultimately, your sex life will be most enhanced if you can talk openly with your lover. But if you need some support toward that goal, you can get it.

Body Image

Having considered your general attitudes about sex, let's now explore your feelings and attitudes about your body. Your body image is your subjective concept of your physical appearance. It includes both how you see your body and how you feel about what you see. People form their body image partly on self-observation and partly on the reactions of others. Your body image may or may not be aligned with objective measurements. A person suffering from anorexia, for example, may perceive her emaciated body to be grotesquely fat.

A culture's standards of attractiveness exert a strong influence over how most people feel about their bodies. We are taught that certain features and dimensions are attractive and others are not. These lessons are constantly reinforced by images in the mass media. In reality, however, even these cultural standards are subjective. Ideal body prototypes vary from decade to decade and century to century. Even individual people of the same culture and time period vary widely in their perception of what is attractive to them. Thus, it is safe to conclude that there is no body type or physical look that is inherently more beautiful than another.

Consider these questions pertaining to your body image:

- How important are looks to you?
- How do you feel about how you look?
- Do you look at yourself in the mirror and like what you see?

- Do you ever wish something were different about your facial features?
- Do you wish you weighed more or less?
- Do you wish you looked stronger, leaner, or more shapely?

It is your birthright to feel and know yourself as beautiful. Nobody can take that away from you. If you have lost your ability to perceive yourself as beautiful or if you have never known yourself as beautiful, you owe it to yourself to find the ability to perceive yourself as such. If you do not feel good about your body or are ashamed of what you see when you look in the mirror, it may be hard to allow another person to see and appreciate your body and give you pleasure. And it may even inhibit your own enjoyment of your body. Chances are, you are your own worst critic when it comes to how you look. While you can't always change what you look like, you can change how you feel about how you look.

Good Overall Health

Does your overall health affect your orgasms? You betcha! It's great to become sex-positive and shame-free, love your body, and be open-minded to all your sexual potential. But without overall good health, your body-mind instrument will not be well tuned. In other words, the more you keep your body healthy and functioning properly, the more it can sing out its gloriousness.

An Orgasmic Diet

Your diet is perhaps the first frontier in improving your overall health. What and how you eat affects not only your digestive system, but also your entire body-mind, including your orgasms. The food you take into your body feeds your nervous and endocrine systems, the two most important systems involved in your orgasms. If you give your body the nourishment it needs for optimal health, you will reap its rewards in orgasmic bliss. Start paying attention to how your food affects your mood, as well as your sex life.

What you eat prior to having sex can also have a direct effect on your sexual experiences. Eating too much or too soon before sex can preoccupy your body with digestion and divert attention from sensual pleasure. The best meal prior to sex would be one that can help you sustain your energy for several hours, without bogging you down or causing wide fluctuations in your blood sugar levels. Try a meal with a good source of protein and fresh vegetables. Stay away from sugar and starchy foods that your body will burn too quickly, leaving you depleted before your sexual fun is over.

 Essential

In her book *The Orgasmic Diet*, Marrena Lindberg identifies several *orgasm killers* that can hamper the body's optimal sexual and orgasmic functioning. Her list includes caffeine, tobacco, sugar, too much soy, omega-6 oils, and trans fats. Watch your intake of these substances and pay attention to how they affect your sexuality.

Staying Fit

Staying fit with regular exercise is also key to sustaining and enjoying a more fulfilling sex life. Good sex is not only about well-functioning genitals. In fact, many of the blocks to vibrant sex as people age reside in other parts of the body. You have more options in sex, for instance, if you have a strong, flexible spine. Certain sexual positions require good arm or leg strength. Sustained sexual encounters require good cardiovascular health and endurance. The more energy you put into keeping your body fit, the more it can reward you with the capacity for vigorous sexual satisfaction.

Regular exercise does more than just keep you in shape. There are numerous other benefits as well. Exercise helps to relax tense muscles, allowing you to better luxuriate in soft, sensual sex. Staying fit also helps with overall relaxation, which can help you sleep better. And since being too tired is one of the most common reasons to miss out on sex, better sleep may directly improve your love life.

Most importantly, regular exercise increases testosterone levels. Testosterone is a hormone that is known to have a strong impact on the human sex drive. In fact, doctors prescribe testosterone to some women as a treatment for a low libido. Exercise naturally increases testosterone levels, while improving just about every other system in your body.

Many people report noticeable increases in sexual desire, activity, and enjoyment simply as a result of beginning to exercise regularly. Integrate this habit into your life and notice a big shift in your overall mood and enjoyment of sex.

Here are some tips on how to safely bring aerobic activity into your daily life:

- Choose an activity that you find enjoyable and that does not cause you any pain.
- Start out at a slow, comfortable, and steady pace.
- Increase your workout's intensity and duration in stages in order to reap the greatest benefits with the fewest risks.
- Plan a workout schedule you know you can adhere to.
- Maximize your comfort and safety by selecting quality equipment and attire for the activity.
- Encourage your lover, friends, or family to join you.
- Challenge yourself by setting reasonable short and long-term goals, and celebrate every success along the way.

Stress Reduction

Accumulated stress can affect your overall mood greatly and take a toll on your sex life. It's hard to enjoy sex when you can't relax. Unfortunately, many people live very stressful lives. Their bodies are constantly in a state of alertness that biologists call the *fight or flight response*, the body's reaction to a perceived danger or threat. During this reaction, hormones such as cortisol and adrenalin are released. These cause the heart to speed up and digestion to slow, redirecting blood flow to major muscle groups and giving the body a burst of energy and strength, preparing it to be able to fight or run away when faced with danger. This response is normally followed by the relaxation response, which returns all systems to normal.

In modern life, however, the fight or flight response is often activated in countless daily activities such as driving, parenting, being a student, earning a living, dealing with bosses and co-workers, and paying the bills. Many people live their lives bombarded by stressful situations and encounters, and the relaxation response has a hard time keeping up with all of the demands. Depending on the number and degree of stressful situations in your life, you may have accumulated stress in your body-mind. Sometimes people are so accustomed to being in a state of fight or flight that they are not even aware of their high levels of background stress.

 Alert

Don't let stress get in the way of your orgasms! Stress affects your libido and has an impact on your hormonal and neurotransmitter levels. If you are having difficulty with orgasms, stress could be the reason. Monitor your ability to orgasm and take steps to reduce stress in your life.

Sadly, people often resort to relieving stress in unhealthy ways. In the long run, this ends up doing more harm than good. Habits like drinking and smoking may feel relaxing, but they actually make your body work harder to maintain its health. Fortunately, there are many healthy habits you can develop to help you reduce and eliminate stress. It is definitely worth your while to explore the options.

Quiet Your Mind

Because your body and mind are so closely connected, quieting your mind can have a profound effect on your body. There are many ways to achieve this, so some exploration may be necessary to find the practices that work the best for you. Meditation is one very effective way to quiet the mind. Meditation relaxes the mind and nervous system through stillness. In meditation, you learn to stay in the present moment with your present experience. When done successfully, mediation induces a deeply relaxed state of being. This can carry over into sexual enjoyment by way of an increased ability to stay focused on your subtle bodily sensations, as well as the present moment interactions you have with your lover.

Sensory Awareness

Sensory awareness practice is a particular type of meditation. In sensory awareness, the mind is focused on all the subtle sensations your body can perceive by being in a relaxed state. To try it, simply lie down somewhere quiet and open all your senses—sight, sound, smell, taste, and touch. It requires getting out of your thoughts and into your body. It requires slowing down, quieting down, and listening acutely but in a relaxed manner. Closing your eyes can help you pay better attention to your other senses.

> **EXERCISE:** Lie down on your back in a warm room. Take several deep breaths and allow your body to relax and melt into the floor. Bring your awareness into your whole body. Become aware of where your body touches the ground. Let yourself feel your clothing touching your skin. Notice areas in your body that are particularly relaxed or tight, warm or cold.

Learning to focus on your physical sensations through a sensory awareness practice can have a profound effect on your sexuality. The more you are able to dial into the subtleties of your experience, the more pleasure you will experience in your sexual encounters.

Yoga

Hatha yoga or any similar stretching practice can also provide multiple benefits to your general health and your enjoyment of sex. Stretching muscles helps them relax and maintains flexibility. If sitting still in meditation or sensory awareness is not relaxing for you, try stretching or yoga instead. You can either quiet your mind to relax your body or relax your body to quiet your mind.

Freeing Your Breath

Have you ever paid attention to your breathing? The breath has a tremendous effect on your body-mind. That's why meditation, yoga, and almost every other relaxation practice involves some amount of focus on your breathing. If your breathing is shallow, it is possible that you are experiencing contraction or tightness in your chest and not getting enough oxygen to optimally support your body and your brain. You may have been breathing this way for so long that you don't notice anything different. Bringing more awareness to your breath and then focusing on deepening and expanding it will help oxygenate your blood, which will in turn lift your mood and improve the functioning of your whole body. Also, the deeper your breath, the greater your capacity for orgasm. Focusing on the breath is an important aspect of some of the enhanced orgasm practices that are discussed in Chapter 14.

Soothe Your Body

Your body sometimes needs help to relax. When you just can't or don't want to do it yourself, you can try using alternative healing practices such as massage, chiropractic techniques, and acupuncture. Each of these can contribute to the well-being of the body-mind and enhance your ability to relax into sex. When your body feels good, your energy is more likely to be open and receptive to erotic pleasure. These healing practices work with your energy in a way that invites more pleasurable sensations in.

Regardless of your chosen method, slowing down can sometimes be a challenge in modern culture. It can be hard to break away from the frenzy and flurry that is all around you. But there is a great reward in letting yourself rest with consciousness. If you pay attention to your senses, you can let them teach you and guide you to more pleasurable experiences. If your lifestyle is keeping you stressed out, consider these questions:

- How much of your life is devoted to work and productivity?
- How much is devoted to relaxation and pleasure?
- Is getting a good night's sleep the extent of your rest?
- Do you pack your vacation time full of activity?
- Do you keep yourself forever busy?
- When you do slow down, do you plop yourself in front of the television or immerse yourself in a magazine, book, crossword puzzle, or newspaper?
- How much time do you spend just listening to your body and paying attention to your senses?

If you find that you don't allow yourself much relaxation time, then you may be missing out on a key ingredient to enjoying your body's full potential for sexual pleasure. To remedy this, consider what changes you might make to your lifestyle that could help you better enjoy yourself, as well as be better prepared for satisfying sex.

A Strong Pelvic Floor

Having emphasized the importance of developing sex-positive attitudes, good health, and the ability to relax accumulated stress, you are now ready to fine-tune one of the most vital and often overlooked muscles in your body. The tone of your pelvic floor can make all the difference in how you experience sex and orgasm.

The muscles of the pelvic floor, particularly the PC muscle (short for *pubococcygeus*), are integral in achieving and enjoying sexual arousal and satisfying orgasms. The PC muscle, also sometimes referred to as the *love muscle* or *sex muscle*, is responsible for supporting the sexual and reproductive organs, as well as the urethra and the rectum. It aids in the start and stop of the flow of urine and bowel movements, helps keep the bladder from leaking, and allows the passage of newborn infants in vaginal births.

Both men and women can benefit from strengthening and toning their PC muscles. Strengthening and toning the pelvic floor will help maintain the integrity of the pelvic floor muscles and tendons, and keep the tissue vital by increasing the blood flow to the pelvic area. It will also increase your awareness of the sensations in your pelvis and allow for greater sensitivity.

 Fact

In 1952, a gynecologist named Dr. Arnold Kegel developed exercises to strengthen the pelvic floor muscles in women who were suffering from urinary incontinence after childbirth. These original PC exercises were named Kegels. Kegel's patients soon discovered another benefit to the strengthening and toning of their pelvic floor muscles—better orgasms.

During arousal and orgasm, the PC muscle contracts involuntarily, initially triggered by direct stimulation or by sexual thoughts and feelings. Once the PC muscle begins its rhythmic pulsations, a positive feedback loop is created. The PC muscle contractions send new arousal messages to the brain. This increased arousal, in turn, causes more pulsations, which sends even more arousal signals to the brain.

Increased Sexual Pleasure and Control

Perhaps the most gratifying and motivating aspect of a strong pelvic floor is increased sexual pleasure. When the PC muscle is well toned, it is able to contract and relax more, helping to build more arousal and intensify sexual sensations. But a stronger PC muscle also increases one's ability to control orgasms, meaning that you can learn to orgasm or not orgasm when you choose. With a strong pelvic floor, men can learn to orgasm without ejaculating by squeezing the PC muscle right before the moment of ejaculatory inevitability. Consequently, they are able to have multiple orgasms. Strengthening the PC muscle can also help women have multiple orgasms and possibly even experience female ejaculation.

It is also believed that men can achieve stronger erections by strengthening the pelvic floor muscles. A stronger erection has the potential to increase pleasure for all parties involved. Likewise, more tone in the pelvic muscles of women can enhance not only her pleasure, but his too.

Finding Your PC Muscle

The PC muscle attaches to your pubic bone (the "P") and your tailbone or coccyx (the "C"). It surrounds the genitals in a figure eight and creates a sling. To locate it and palpate it on your body, place the tips of your fingers of one hand into the fleshy part just above your pubic bone, which is above your genitals and near the top of your pubic hair. Then place the tips of your fingers of the other hand on the underside of your tailbone, which is at the bottom of your spine near the top of your crack. Now squeeze the muscles of your pelvic floor as if you were trying to stop your urine mid-flow. The muscle you feel being engaged is your PC muscle.

Pelvic Floor Exercises

There are two basic ways to exercise your PC muscle—one is to squeeze and lift the muscle on its own. You can vary the duration of time you squeeze and the amount of time you relax between squeezes. The alternative way, for women only, is to insert an object, such as a kegelcisor, into the vagina and squeeze and lift the object.

Start out with 10–15 repetitions a few times a day. Be sure to relax all the way after each squeeze. The relaxation phase is just as important, if not more, as the squeezing phase. A PC muscle may be strong, but it is not well toned if it cannot relax as well as contract. With or without an inserted object, proceed by lifting and squeezing the PC muscle on your exhale and relaxing on your inhale. Breathe deeply and slowly. Do not get frustrated with yourself if you are having difficulty isolating your PC muscle. This takes time and practice. As you get stronger, you can increase the number of repetitions, but remember to continue to relax in between squeezing.

 Alert

Whichever version of the exercise you choose, the important thing to remember is to start out slow. You can overwork and strain your PC muscle, just like the other muscles in your body. Take the time to gradually build up the strength in your pelvic floor, slowly increasing the number of repetitions and duration of these exercises.

Your body-mind is a fabulous instrument capable of playing beautiful music indeed. But it needs your help to stay well tuned. Clearing out any shame you may feel about sex or your body, attending to your general health and fitness, learning how to relax and tune into your physical sensations, and strengthening the muscles of your pelvic floor will help you prepare yourself for some of the most orgasmic concerts of your life!

CHAPTER 3

The Do Re Mi of Orgasm

A n orgasm is the amazing result of many anatomical structures and physiological systems working together. Enjoyable
orgasms are like well-played music. They involve all the basic parts
of your instrument playing in harmony. Unfortunately, many people begin having sex with very little background knowledge about
how their body or their partner's body works. This can sometimes
lead to frustrating experiences. For more reliably satisfying sex, it is
helpful to know all the different sexual body parts and understand
what notes they play.

Her Sexual Anatomy

Understanding your sexual anatomy will help you learn how to better pleasure yourself and communicate with partners about how
they can pleasure you. Women, in particular, have been histori-
cally in the dark about their sexual organs, partly because of the
cultural taboo about masturbation and touching their genitals and
partly because of the placement of their genitalia on their bodies.
Women's vulvas are tucked away and difficult to see, and women
do not have the benefit of having their genitals all out in the open,
or the explicit permission to touch their genitalia as boys and men
do in order to urinate.

Many people refer to the female genitalia globally as the vagina. In actuality, however, the vagina is only one part of a woman's genitals. Women have both external and internal sexual organs.

The Vulva, the External Female Genitalia

The part of the female genitalia that is visible from the outside is called the vulva. Vulvas come in many different colors, shapes, and sizes. Indeed, no two are alike. There is really no such thing as normal when it comes to vulvas, so there is no need to be concerned or distressed about how yours looks. Just learn to appreciate your vulva's unique beauty and all of the pleasure it has in store for you. The different parts of the vulva are the pubic mound, the outer and inner labia, the vestibule, the vaginal opening, the urethral opening, the greater vestibular glands, the perineum, and the clitoris and clitoral hood.

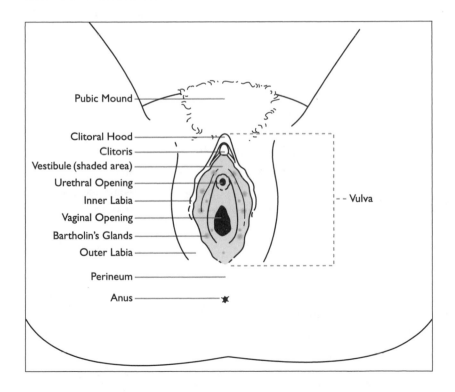

The Pubic Mound

The pubic mound, also known as the mons pubis, is the soft mound of fatty tissue that covers the pubic bone at the top of the vulva. It contains many nerves. After the onset of puberty, it becomes covered with pubic hair. The pubic mound provides a structurally strong, cushioned surface for the bumping and grinding sex often involves.

The Outer Labia

Below the pubic mound are the softer vulva tissues. Surrounding this area are the outer vaginal lips or outer labia. They are the two outer mounds of spongy flesh on either side of the vaginal opening. They are generally covered in pubic hair. The clinical term for these lips, *labia majora*, is Latin for larger lips, but some vulvas have inner lips that are actually larger than the outer ones. The outer labia cover and protect the more delicate inner parts of the female genitals.

The Inner Labia

Resting inside the outer labia are the inner vaginal lips or inner labia (Latin: *labia minora*). The inner labia extend from the clitoris around either side of the urethral and vaginal openings. In some women the inner labia are completely concealed within the outer labia, but in others they protrude. Inner labia are sensitive, delicate, hairless lips. They are made up of erectile tissue, so they can become engorged during sexual arousal.

The Vestibule

The vestibule is the part of the vulva that is inside the inner labia. The term actually means a hall or lobby adjacent to the entrance of a building. The urethra, the greater vestibular glands, and the vagina all open into the vestibule.

The Urethral Opening

At the head of the vestibule is the urethral opening. The urethra is the tube that connects your bladder to the outside of your body, enabling you to discharge urine. Although its function is not reproductive, it is often considered part of the genitalia because of its location.

The Bartholin's Glands

There are two glands located slightly below and on either side of the vaginal opening. These are called the Bartholin's glands, also known as the greater vestibular glands. They are responsible for secreting mucus when a woman is sexually aroused, providing lubrication that will assist in intercourse or any other kind of penetration. The greater vestibular glands are the female version of the Cowper's glands in the male.

The Vaginal Opening

The vaginal opening (Latin: the *introitus*) is the narrowest portion of the vagina, located at the base of the vestibule. At birth, the vaginal opening in most women is partially covered by a thin membrane known as the hymen, which varies greatly in size and thickness.

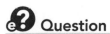 Question

If a girl or woman does not have a hymen, is she technically not a virgin?
Traditionally, a young woman's virginity was sometimes confirmed by checking to see if she had an intact hymen. The hymen, however, can be broken or dissolved in a number of ways, and its nonexistence does not necessarily mean a woman has lost her virginity. Hymens can rupture as a result of some strenuous physical activity, insertion of a tampon during menstruation, or any form of vaginal penetration.

The Perineum

At the rear or bottom of the vulva is the perineum. The perineum is the conglomeration of muscles situated between and around the anus and vagina. These muscles help support the pelvic cavity and keep the pelvic organs in place. The skin in this area is rich in nerves and therefore sensitive to the touch.

The Clitoris

Within the vulva lies the magnificent clitoris. The clitoris is perhaps the greatest gem of sexual pleasure in a woman. In fact, the sole function of the clitoris is to provide sexual arousal. Some people consider the existence of the clitoris to be proof positive that humans were made to enjoy sexual pleasure.

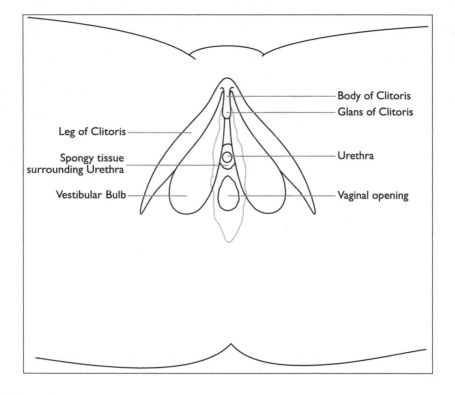

The clitoris has many more parts to it than most people realize. It is formed from the same type of tissues that form the penis in males, so many of the parts have corollaries in the penis. Overall, there is an abundance of nerve endings throughout the clitoris and in the area surrounding it, making this area extremely sensitive to direct and indirect pressure and touch. The clitoris consists of the hood, glans, shaft, crura, and vestibular bulbs. The specific size and shape of these parts of the clitoris vary significantly from woman to woman.

The Hood

The clitoris is covered and protected by a fold of tissue that is part of the inner labia, making up what is called a clitoral hood, or prepuce. This hood is somewhat similar to the foreskin of the penis.

The Glans

Aside from the hood, the only part of the clitoris that is visible from the outside is the glans or head. The glans is either tucked under, peaks out, or protrudes out from underneath the clitoral hood. It looks like a small, shiny button. It is by far the most sensitive part of the clitoris, hosting the greatest number of nerve endings per square inch. It is analogous to the glans or head of the penis.

The Shaft

The shaft, or the body, is approximately one to two inches long and a little over half an inch wide. It contains two spongy erectile bodies of tissue called cavernous bodies, or the corpora cavernosa. This tissue becomes engorged (fills with blood) when a woman becomes sexually aroused, increasing the size of the clitoris. The shaft of the clitoris is analogous with the shaft of the penis in the male.

The Crura

The base of the shaft of the clitoris attaches to the pubic bone and then divides into the two legs, or crura, which are each between two and four inches long. The legs of the clitoris follow and attach to the arch of the pubic bone. The crura also contain the spongy erectile tissue cavernous bodies.

Vestibular Bulbs

The vestibular bulbs, also called the clitoral bulbs, consist of two masses of spongy erectile tissue on either side of the vestibule. They are joined in the front by a narrow band called the pars intermedia. The vestibular bulbs swell with blood during sexual arousal, making the vaginal opening smaller, which increases the gripping and hugging of a penis or any other penetrating object.

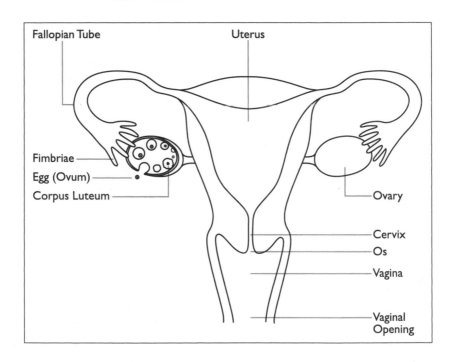

The Internal Female Genitalia

The internal female genitalia make up the main part of the reproductive anatomy of a woman. This includes the ovaries, the fallopian tubes, the uterus, the cervix, the vagina, the Skene's glands, and the urethral sponge. Most of the internal female genitalia are impossible to see. With the help of a speculum, a flashlight, and a mirror, however, you can get a glance at the vaginal walls and the cervix.

The Ovaries

Human eggs are produced and stored in the ovaries, which also serve as the glands that produce female sex hormones. Women generally have two ovaries. They are almond-shaped, measure about one and a half inches long, and are situated at the end of the fallopian tubes on either side of the uterus. The ovaries alternate the task of maturing and releasing one egg per month.

The Fallopian Tubes

The fallopian tubes are the four-inch tunnels through which an egg travels from the ovary to the uterus. As a method of permanent birth control, some women get their tubes tied (surgically blocked) so that eggs can no longer make their way to the uterus, thus preventing pregnancy.

The Uterus

The uterus, also referred to as the womb, is the organ that has the potential to be a home for a developing infant. It is about the size and shape of a small upside down pear. It consists of three layers of tissue. The inner layer, the lining of the uterus, is called the endometrium. This is the layer that either helps support and nurture a developing infant or sloughs off during menstruation if no fertilized egg has implanted itself. The middle layer, called the myometrium, is a very powerful muscle that extends in all directions. This is the muscle that stretches to accommodate a growing fetus and also contracts strongly enough during childbirth so that the baby can make its way out of the womb. The outer layer, called the perimetrium, is a thin membrane that encases the outer part of the uterus.

The Cervix

The cervix is the tip of the uterus that can be felt at the back of the vagina. It is made up of very strong muscles and has no nerve endings on its surface. The opening in the center of the cervix is called the os. It is through the os that sperm enter the uterus and menstrual blood exits the uterus. In childbirth, an infant can pass through a greatly dilated os to the vaginal canal.

The Vagina

The vagina is made up of extremely expandable tissue, which forms a canal, about four inches long, extending into the body and angling upward toward the small of the back. It is considered a potential space. Most of the time, its tissues rest against themselves. It expands only during high states of arousal or childbirth. The tissue of the outer third of the vagina is comprised of numerous ridges and folds. This outer third has more nerve endings than the rest of the vagina and is consequently the most sensitive portion. The tissue of the inner two-thirds of the vagina is much smoother. It is less sensitive to light touch, friction, or vibration, but it is still very responsive to pressure. The vagina has many functions: One is to allow for penetration for pleasure or procreation, another is to carry menstrual flow out of the body, and another is to serve as a birth canal.

The Skene's Glands

The Skene's glands, also known as the lesser vestibular or para-urethral glands, are located on the anterior wall of the vagina, near the lower end of the urethra. They vary in size from one woman to another and appear to be missing altogether in some women.

The Skene's glands are the female version of the prostate gland in males. They produce a clear or milky fluid that is similar to the fluid the prostate generates in males. In women who ejaculate, this fluid is released into urethral tract and expelled from the urethral opening. Because of the similarities, many researchers are beginning to refer to the Skene's glands as the female prostate. The location of the Skene's glands is also known as the G-spot (the Grafenberg spot) and the general area is that of the urethral sponge.

 Alert

Douching or using feminine deodorant sprays is unnecessary and perhaps even harmful. The vagina cleans itself and does not need help from commercial products. The perfumes and chemicals used in commercial products can irritate the delicate tissues of the vagina and even cause vaginal infections. Simply shower to remove any unwanted natural discharge or odor.

The Urethral Sponge

The urethral sponge is the spongy cushion of erectile tissue surrounding the urethra. During arousal, it becomes engorged with blood and compresses the urethra, helping to prevent urination during sexual activity.

His Sexual Anatomy

While a man's sexual anatomy is a lot more out in the open than a woman's, there is still a lot that men may not understand about their genitals and how they function. Learning more about your sexual anatomy can help you expand your awareness of the many possibilities for sexual pleasure that may yet be undiscovered. Just as that of women, male sexual anatomy can also be divided into internal and external genitalia.

The External Male Genitalia

The external male genitals consist of the penis, the scrotum, and the urethral opening. You are probably aware of this much, but you may lack knowledge of the more intricate details of this part of your anatomy and its physiology.

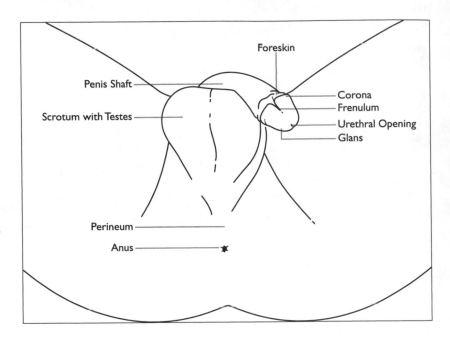

The Penis

The penis is the main source of sexual pleasure for males. It is made up of three columns of spongy erectile tissue—two corpora cavernosa or cavernous bodies and one corpus spongiosum or spongy body. These columns become engorged, or filled with blood, when a man is sexually aroused, making the penis erect. This prepares the penis for intercourse or any other penetration.

The penis is made up of several different parts, each of which has its own unique capacity for sexual arousal and pleasure. These parts include the head or glans, the urethral opening, the foreskin, the corona, the frenulum, and the shaft.

The Glans

The glans or head of the penis is the rounded part at the end of the shaft. It is a highly sensitive area with many nerve endings. The glans of the penis is developed out of the same tissue as that of the glans of the clitoris. At the tip of the glans is the urethral opening where urine expels itself from the body.

 Essential

Penises come in all shapes and sizes. The size of a penis, in nearly all cases, has nothing to do with how a penis functions or the pleasurable sensations it is capable of experiencing. When it comes to providing pleasure, it is the fit that counts, not the size.

The Foreskin

The foreskin, or prepuce, is the double-layered fold of skin that covers the glans in a flaccid penis. It is like the clitoral hood that covers and protects the clitoris on the female. The foreskin retracts to just below the glans when the penis is erect. It protects the glans and the frenulum, keeping these tissues lubricated and shielded from abrasion or injury. Many men have had their foreskins removed when they were infants in a process called circumcision. In circumcised men, the glans is therefore exposed at all times.

The Frenulum

The frenulum is the indentation found on the underside of the penis where the glans and the shaft meet. The frenulum is a highly sensitive area for most men.

The Corona

The corona, sometimes called the coronal ridge, is the ridged band that separates the head of the penis from the shaft. It is a highly innervated smooth muscle that radiates from the frenulum and surrounds the inner tip of the foreskin. It contains approximately 80 percent of the male erogenous tissue and is extremely sensitive to light touch, stretching, folding, pressure, and temperature. When the foreskin is pulled back, the ridged band lies just behind the crest of the glans.

The Shaft of the Penis

The shaft is the part of the penis that extends out from the body to the head of the penis. When it is flaccid, the skin on the shaft is loose and stretchy. Unlike the skin everywhere else on the body that attaches to the underlying tissues, the foreskin and the skin on the shaft are loose and can glide freely along the shaft of the penis, which reduces friction and abrasion and keeps the lubricating fluid flowing during stimulation, intercourse, or other penetration.

 Alert

Sensitivity of the various parts of the penis and testicles varies significantly from man to man. For example, even though many people consider the shaft of the penis to be less sensitive than the glans, some men have highly sensitive areas on the shafts of their penises.

The Scrotum

The scrotum, or scrotal sac, is a thin-walled muscular pouch that has two compartments to house the testicles and is located underneath the penis. One of its functions is to maintain the testicles at a temperature slightly below the rest of the body's temperature. This is achieved through a process known as the cremasteric reflex. This reflex causes the scrotum and testes to pull in closer to the body for more warmth or release further away from the body to cool down.

The Internal Male Genitalia

As in the female, the internal genital structures of the male are primarily concerned with reproduction. The internal genital organs or structures are the testicles, the urethra, the epididymis, the vas deferens, the seminal vesicle, the ejaculatory duct, the Cowper's glands, and the prostate.

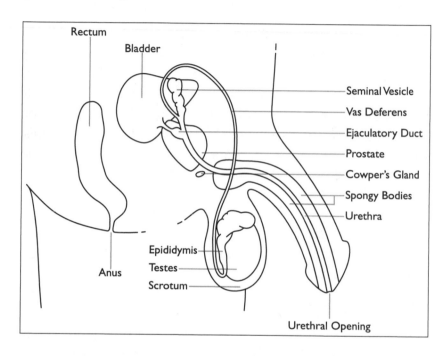

The Testicles

The testicles, also referred to as the testes, produce both sperm and male sex hormones. They are the male counterpart to the female's ovaries. The testicles are contained within the scrotum, or the scrotal sac or pouch. They are usually very sensitive to impact but can also be pleasurably fondled.

The Epididymis

The epididymis is a narrow, tightly coiled tube that connects the back of the testicles to the vas deferens, through which semen flows during ejaculation.

The Vas Deferens

The vas deferens are two ducts that pass above and behind the bladder. They provide temporary storage for sperm and they are responsible for propelling sperm during ejaculation.

The Urethra

The urethra is the last part of the urinary tract, ending at the tip of the penis. Its function is to allow the passage of urine and semen.

The Prostate

The prostate is the gland that surrounds the urethra just below the bladder. When healthy, it is about the size of a walnut. It is responsible for secreting some of the fluids that make up the semen.

The Seminal Vesicles

The seminal vesicles are a pair of glands located behind the bladder in the male. They are responsible for secreting a large portion of the fluid that ultimately becomes semen.

The Ejaculatory Ducts

The ejaculatory ducts are the channels that join the vas deferens and the seminal vesicles. They pass through the prostate gland and drain into the urethra. During ejaculation, the semen passes through these ducts and out of the body through the penis.

The Cowper's Glands

The Cowper's or bulbourethral glands are two small, rounded bodies about the size of peas, located behind the urethra. They are responsible for secreting a clear, pre-ejaculatory fluid, generated upon sexual arousal. They are the male equivalent to the Bartholin's glands in females.

Human Sexual Response

Having covered the main components of sexual anatomy, it is time to take a look at the sequence of physiological events that happen during sex. When aroused, either through mental or physical stimulation, both male and female bodies undergo a series of changes. From an evolutionary perspective, many of these changes function to prepare male and female bodies for coitus, or vaginal intercourse. Of course, how you respond to these physiological changes and the behaviors that you choose to participate in are completely your own choice.

 Fact

The laboratory research of Masters and Johnson, which began in the 1950s, involved observing the sexual response cycle of 382 women and 312 men, ranging in age from eighteen to eighty-nine. The research studied more than 10,000 complete sexual response cycles. This research provided some of the first data pertaining to the anatomy and physiology of the human sexual response.

The Sexual Response Cycle

The sequence of physiological events that make up the human sexual response was first identified by the pioneering research of Dr. William Masters and Virginia Johnson. Masters and Johnson called this sequence "the sexual response cycle." In their work, they identified four distinct stages of sexual response: excitement, plateau, orgasm, and resolution. Subsequent researchers have added a fifth stage, desire, which comes before the excitement stage.

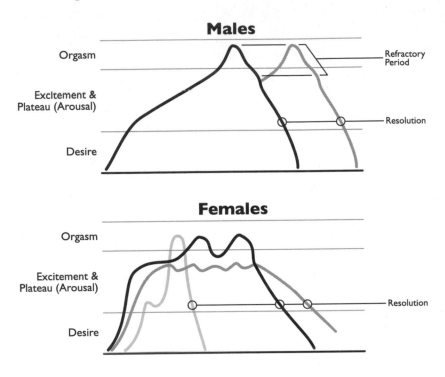

Stage 1: Desire

The initial stage in the sexual response cycle for men and women is desire, the urge for sexual intimacy or sexual gratification. Desire takes place mostly in the mind. It is related to your sex drive or libido. It could be considered the potential for sexual arousal or excitement. There are many cues that incite sexual desire; some are physical, others are psychological. These cues may come in a variety of stimuli. Here are some examples:

- Visual: The appearance of a particular person or some physically appealing aspect or attribute of that person, or a beautiful landscape or sunset.

- Auditory: The sound of someone's voice, sighs, moans, or breathing, or a beautiful song.
- Olfactory: The smell of someone's body odor or perfume, or the scent of honeysuckle on the breeze.
- Kinesthetic: Physical activity, dancing, running, yoga, or another type of movement.
- Tactile: The feel of someone's soft skin, firm muscles, soft cotton or silk, or warm water.
- Memory: The recollection of an old lover or erotic encounter.
- Fantasy: The image of some romantic or erotic interlude with someone you know, have just met, or have never seen before.

What gets your desire going is highly individualistic and is based on a variety of factors, including your hormone levels, your connection to a partner, your life experiences, and the sexual cues in your environment. Desire can be adversely affected by many factors as well, including poor health, low self-esteem, high stress levels, low energy, shame, or concerns about health risks. It is important to note that you may feel desire without any object of desire, just a feeling of wanting sexual gratification.

Essential

For some people, the desire phase may seem intricately woven with the excitement phase. There may be very little perceivable distinction between the two. Although it is possible that you could be completely unaware of the desire phase, without it there would be no excitement phase.

Stage 2: Excitement

The second stage in the sexual response cycle is that of excitement. It is also called the arousal phase. This is the stage where you start to sense erotic feelings and responses in your body. The onset of the excitement phase varies from person to person due to a variety of factors. An adolescent boy, for example, may enter into the excitement phase with very little physical or mental stimulation. Older women, on the other hand, may need significant physical stimulation, fantasy, and intimacy in order to become fully aroused. Though the time and effort it takes to enter the excitement phase varies greatly, the majority of physiological changes that take place are the same, varying only in degree.

During this phase there is an increase in heart rate, blood flow, breathing, and muscle tension. The increase in blood flow increases the body's overall warmth and may cause a "sex flush" or flushed skin, particularly on the face, the abdomen and the chest. This can happen in both genders, although it is more common in women. There is also an increase in sensitivity to stimulation and a reduction in sensitivity to pain. The nipples may become erect in both men and women, and many involuntary and voluntary muscles begin contracting.

The excitement phase also initiates the important processes of genital vasoconstriction and genital vasocongestion. In genital vasoconstriction, the veins carrying blood away from the genitals become narrow, restricting the flow of blood leaving the genital tissues. This allows for genital vasocongestion, also called engorgement, which is the pooling of blood into the genital tissues. These processes are what make the penis erect and the clitoris, vagina, and vulva swell.

In women, a few other changes occur during the excitement phase. Breasts may increase in size and the vaginal walls become lubricated. The vagina lengthens, the upper portion of the vagina balloons, or widens, the uterus rises, and the labia swell and separate. In men, the penis becomes erect, the scrotum thickens and the testicles rise up closer to the body.

Stage 3: Plateau

The third stage of the sexual response cycle is the plateau stage. In the plateau stage, you are sustaining a very high level of arousal. This stage is usually brought on by continuous physical stimulation of specific erogenous zones, which may be supplemented by mental stimulation, such as fantasy. This is the state you are in just before orgasm, although this state may come and go numerous times before orgasm occurs. In other words, you may reach a plateau for a stretch of time and then drop back down to a lower level of arousal before rising up again.

During this stage, all of the physiological changes that took place in the arousal phase intensify and there is a sense of impending orgasm. Muscle tension, breathing, pulse rates, and blood pressure increase further. You may have muscle spasms in your feet, face, or hands.

In this stage women experience what is known as the orgasmic platform. The lower third of the vagina becomes even more engorged, tightening and narrowing that portion of the vagina. The uterus elevates fully, and the walls of the upper two-thirds of the vagina expand even more, creating a tenting effect. Lubrication increases, nipples become larger, and the labia darken in color. The clitoris becomes highly sensitive and retracts under the clitoral hood.

In men, the penis becomes fully erect to the limits of its capacity; the testicles become engorged and are 50 percent larger than they were during non-arousal. The glans of the penis swells fully. The Cowper's glands may secrete pre-ejaculatory fluid, which may contain some sperm.

Stage 4: Orgasm

The fourth stage of the sexual response cycle is the orgasm, or climax. It occurs at the peak of the plateau phase. It is characterized by involuntary muscle contractions of the pelvic regions in men and women and a sudden release of sexual tension. The body releases chemicals called endorphins, which create intensely pleasurable sensations throughout the whole body. It is generally the shortest of all the phases. It is usually, but not always, accompanied by ejaculation of semen in the male and, more rarely, ejaculation of fluids in the female.

 Alert

Sexual arousal and activity does not always culminate in orgasm, nor does it need to. Achieving orgasm requires a number of factors or conditions to be in place, and not all sexual encounters satisfy these conditions. Sometimes orgasm is not even the goal of a particular sexual activity. It's your choice whether you want the sex you have to lead to orgasm.

Stage 5: Resolution

The fifth and final stage of the sexual response cycle is resolution. This is the stage wherein all of the body's systems return to normal. The heartbeat and breathing slow back down and the muscles relax. Vasocongestion is released and the blood flows back to the rest of the body.

Refractory Period

The refractory period is the time it takes after one orgasm for the body to experience another orgasm. This period varies among individuals and between genders. Men generally have a longer refractory period than women. Women with short refractory periods are capable of experiencing multiple orgasms. Some men may be able to experience multiple orgasms as well. If a man learns to orgasm without ejaculation, then he may be able to reduce his refractory period and maintain his erection between orgasms.

The Body Systems Involved in Sexual Arousal and Orgasm

Although the sexual response cycle is laid out as a progression of bodily events, there are actually many different systems working together simultaneously. These systems are intricately woven together, responding to cues and messages sent between them to keep the process of arousal moving along. The body systems involved in sexual arousal and orgasm are the nervous system, the cardiovascular system, the exocrine glands, the muscular-skeletal system, and the endocrine system.

The Involuntary Nervous System

Sexual response is initially triggered by your nervous system perceiving some form of erotic stimulation, either mental or physical. Physical stimulation may be sensations of touch on or near your erogenous zones, be it either the genitals or some other sensitive part of your body. Mental stimulation may come in the form of erotic thoughts or fantasy, or it may involve mentally focusing on your erogenous zones and the possibility of pleasurable sensations there.

The nervous system responds in multiple ways to this sensory or mental input. The neural impulses communicate with all the other systems in the body. The brain tells certain hormones to begin flowing, certain muscles to begin tightening, and certain glands to begin secreting. Most of this communication is involuntary, like a reflex, and not in your direct control.

The stages of the sexual response cycle involve a steadily increasing activation of the sympathetic nervous system. This involuntary part of the nervous system is what prepares a person for intense activity. Activation of the sympathetic nervous system increases heart rate, breathing rate, blood pressure, and muscular tension, among other effects.

The counterpart of the sympathetic nervous system is the parasympathetic nervous system. The parasympathetic nervous system prepares the body for rest and relaxation. It slows the heart rate and breathing rate and decreases blood pressure and muscle tension.

 Fact

The main nerves that service the pelvic region and sexual organs are the pudenal nerves, the pelvic nerves, the hypogastric nerves, and the vagus nerves. The pudenal nerves are believed to be the main nerves responsible in carrying out the arousal and orgasm messages to and from the brain. They service both the clitoris and the penis.

The intensity of orgasm is partly a result of the dramatic shift in the nervous system that occurs during orgasm. Suddenly, the sympathetic nervous system is deactivated and the parasympathetic nervous system is triggered. Such a dramatic shift in the nervous system results in some of the extraordinary sensations associated with orgasm: simultaneous excitement and release. It also accounts for the peaceful states people often experience after orgasm.

Feedback Loops

Several body systems engage in positive feedback loops as sexual excitement increases. One example of this is vasoconstriction. The brain, in response to some initial stimulation, may tell the cardiovascular system to restrict blood flow out of the genital area. The brain then senses the resulting engorgement as a new source of sexual stimulation. This induces it to direct the veins to constrict even further to maximize the engorgement of sexual tissue.

Another example of a positive feedback loop involves the muscular-skeletal system. Initial stages of arousal result in subtle muscle contractions in the pelvic area. The increased muscular activity heightens sensation in the pelvis, which then feeds the brain with a wealth of sensory stimulation, which in turn focuses the brain on the body and away from distracting thoughts. This increasing stream of sensory input to the nervous system helps create the cascading effect of increasing arousal, potentially leading to orgasm.

Finally, the endocrine system and the nervous system interact in positive feedback loops as well. Researchers have not yet uncovered all the details of the interplay between hormones and the brain, but they do know that certain hormones can increase or decrease the threshold for the excitation of nerves. Thus, the hormones that the brain directs the gonads (the ovaries and testes) to release end up affecting the type of information the brain subsequently receives. In other words, sexual stimulation results in the release of hormones that keep the brain even more focused on sex.

When you have sex, there's a lot going on behind the scenes. The specific sexual organs are each doing their job. The larger systems of your body are interacting with each other. Each sensation or event builds on the previous ones in a response cycle that may ultimately lead to orgasm. While many of the details of these bodily functions are not consciously directed, it can be helpful to understand the whole picture. Your body is an amazing and complex instrument, inherently capable of great pleasure.

CHAPTER 4

Exploring Your Erotic Body-Mind

Your body is truly a remarkable instrument, capable of astounding erotic pleasure. The more you accept and appreciate all of the feelings, thoughts, and sensations that make up your erotic nature, the more pleasure you will be capable of experiencing. Unfortunately, past experiences or social conditioning may have shut down a part of your sexual aliveness. Openly exploring your own body and your fantasies is a great way to reclaim your inherent right to all of the pleasure your body has available for you.

Accepting Your Sexual Self

Sexual self-acceptance means being okay with the sexual thoughts, fantasies, images, and sexual behaviors that turn you on. Accepting your sexual self is key to allowing arousal and orgasms to move through your body, and to more fully enjoy your erotic potential. Consider the perspective that anything you do, think, or feel to provide yourself with erotic pleasure that does not harm anyone is inherently acceptable. Claim the freedom to enjoy whatever fantasies your mind may have. Open yourself to the pleasure of touch anywhere your body might enjoy it.

Your Own True Authority

In sexual self-acceptance, you embrace your sexuality and identify yourself as the only true authority on your sexuality. Each person's sexuality is a unique combination of all human sexual possibilities. There is no reason to give anyone the power to define what is supposed to be true for you in regard to your sexual needs and desires. Of course, you may not always get your way in any given sexual encounter. Your inherent right to your desires does not mean you can impose them on others without their consent. It does mean, however, that you need never feel wrong or bad for wanting what you want, or for getting turned on by whatever turns you on. You deserve to be proud of your unique sexuality.

Difficulty Accepting Your Sexual Self

You may find that accepting your sexual self is easier in concept than in reality. If so, you are definitely not alone. In most cultures, everyone is exposed to some level of shame about sex. If you find that you judge yourself or worry about yourself for having particular sexual desires or fantasies, it may be worth your while to take a closer look at where these judgments come from.

There are many reasons why you may have difficulty accepting your sexual self. These reasons usually stem from negative messages about sexuality that you got from your family, religion, or a particular culture. Other self-judgments could spring from negative past sexual experiences. You may question your desirability to others. Maybe you do not feel deserving of erotic pleasure. Or perhaps you received very little touch or physical affection as a child, leaving you uncomfortable with touch or physical pleasure even as an adult. It could be that your sexual desires scare you because they are taboo. Whatever the reasons, it may benefit you to do some self-exploration and re-evaluation of some of your attitudes and beliefs about your sexuality.

Early Negative Sexual Experiences

Your first sexual experiences can have a tremendous impact on how you feel about your sexual self. Were your first experiences consensual? Were you judged or shamed? Did you enjoy yourself? Did you have to hide or be secretive? These factors may all influence your feelings about sex, for better or for worse. Fortunately, if you do have painful memories from your sexual past, you do not have to let them continue to interfere with your enjoyment of sexuality today. You can explore and understand the circumstances that surrounded the negative event. In doing so, you can take the power away from any negative memories. Look to your partner, a good friend, or a therapist to assist and support you in this process.

 Essential

> Creative forms of self-expression, such as art, dance, music, or writing, can be a part of your healing path to help you move beyond any painful memories from your sexual past. They can help you get to a place where your past no longer negatively affects your enjoyment of your erotic self.

Negative Messages Pertaining to Sex

From the time you were young, you received messages about sexuality. Unfortunately, many of them were probably negative. It could be that sex was simply never discussed, implying that sex is not something to be talked about. Or perhaps you were told not to touch yourself down there. Most children are raised to believe that sex is dirty and that their genitals are something to avoid. Some are even taught that masturbation is a sin.

As you got older, you were probably exposed to many judgments about specific sexual behaviors. Fear is the root of most of these judgments. The people espousing such negative messages are usually afraid of unbridled sexuality. They may even be afraid of their own sexuality. Thus they seek to repress everyone's sexuality as a way to try to have mastery over their own. If any judgments from others are affecting your enjoyment of your body, perhaps it makes sense to question the motivations of the people who have offered those judgments.

Feeling Undesirable

You may suffer from low sexual self-esteem and feel undesirable. This can greatly affect your sexual self-acceptance. If you can't believe that someone could find you sexually attractive, then you may not accept your sexual urges or feelings, because you are afraid that you will never be able to satisfy them. You may need to do some personal growth work, perhaps with the help of a therapist, in order to begin to increase your sense of desirability and accept your erotic feelings.

Touch Deprived

If you did not receive much touch or affection as a child, you may later feel very uncomfortable with any kind of touch, including sexual affection. Or you may be comfortable with sex but uncomfortable with lots of touch during foreplay. All humans need physical touch to feel safe and connected. People who spurn affection leave this need tragically unmet in themselves. If you did not get much or any touch, you could benefit from doing some healing work in this area. Body-oriented psychotherapy and massage are both good ways to begin to address this issue.

Fear of Sexual Urges, Feelings, and Desires

Sexual urges and feelings are some of the most powerful feelings we can experience as human beings. They can be scary. They are a force to be reckoned with. You may be afraid that you will not be able to control your urges. Or you may be afraid of your desires simply because you do not understand them. Whichever the case, take a close look at the underbelly of your desires.

Face the fears directly. Often by looking more closely, with self-reflection or research, you can alleviate your fears. Talking with a close friend, a clinical sexologist, or a sex therapist is a good way to get some support.

 Fact

> The *attachment theory* postulates that infants and young children need to be held and touched when distressed in order for them to learn how to soothe and calm their own nervous systems. Research in the fields of neuroscience and psychology are finding a significant link between emotional needs getting met in the first years of life and healthy adult relationships.

Your Arousal Map

Who are you sexually? Your arousal map is the constellation of the things that turn you on. It contains all the fantasies and activities you find sexually arousing. Following this map can lead you to orgasm. Your arousal map is unique. You come into life with a particular genetic blueprint. You are raised by a particular family. You are exposed to particular attitudes, habits, and values in a specific community full of its own rules and expected behaviors. As you grow, you have unique experiences and you try to make sense of it all. You start to define your own identity, which may or may not be aligned with your family and community.

Part of your personal identity is your sexual identity, your arousal map. How do you define yourself as an erotic being? Here are some questions that will help you gain more understanding of your unique arousal map:

- When have you felt the most desire or pleasure?
- What places, times of day, or partners have aroused you the most?

- How is your current sexual life similar to or different from your past sexual life?
- What things currently increase or decrease your desire?
- What is the perfect erotic situation for you?

Exploring Sexual Thoughts and Feelings

One way to start exploring your body's response to sexual stimulation is by examining your sexual thoughts and feelings. Some say that the mind is the most erogenous zone of all. Some people report being capable of having an orgasm solely through fantasizing, without any accompanying physical stimulation. If you haven't been using your mind to help get you turned on, then you should consider giving it more focus. This is particularly true if you have any difficulty sustaining arousal or achieving orgasm. Sexual thoughts and feelings come in many forms. Here are a few:

- Being in love or lust and thinking about the object of your desire.
- Mental images of something or someone that turns you on.
- Fantasies of something erotic happening to you.
- Fantasies of witnessing something erotic.
- Anticipating sexual touch by yourself or another.
- Anticipating a sexual encounter with someone you lust after.

EXERCISE: Let your mind wander and welcome any sexual thoughts or feelings. Make a mental note about the nature of each. Are there any recurring themes? What is your emotional reaction to any of your fantasies? Feel free to improvise, creating new mental images or fantasies to add to the images your mind spontaneously creates. See how this influences your overall state of arousal.

Many people inhibit their sexual thoughts and fantasies out of fear. As long as you are able to clearly differentiate fantasy from reality, your sexual thoughts and feelings will not get you into trouble. Actual sexual behaviors, on the other hand, do need careful consideration so that you stay safe and do not endanger others. You may find yourself getting turned on by thoughts or fantasies that you know better than to pursue in reality. This is completely normal. It is very common to get aroused by taboo scenarios or even patently unsafe behaviors. Just because the idea of something turns you on, it does not mean you will ever want or feel compelled to act it out. It is important to remember that when you fantasize, you are not harming yourself or others, so you have a right to enjoy whatever your mind comes up with.

If you find that a fantasy of yours creates icky feelings, you will need to address this so that the uncomfortable feelings won't diminish your sexual arousal. One option is simply to try to avoid focusing on any distressing fantasies. There are limitless ways to become aroused, and if one isn't working for you, you may be able to shift your focus to find another. Bringing your attention to physical sensations might help. Or you might actively create a fantasy that is more comfortable for you.

If you find that you cannot get comfortable with certain fantasies that turn you on, then you may benefit from exploring your uneasiness with a sex therapist. Such exploration may help you get to the root of your discomfort. This might enable you to more easily enjoy the eroticism your fantasies can provide for you. Alternatively, you may discover something in your self-exploration that changes the troubling fantasy or its power to turn you on.

 Alert

If you are afraid of acting on a sexual thought or feeling that would get you into trouble, then you should seek professional help. It is important to recognize when you do not have control over your behavior with regard to certain sexual thoughts and feelings.

Getting Up Close and Personal

Knowing how your body likes to be touched is an important part of knowing yourself and getting in touch with your sexuality. You learned about your sexual anatomy in Chapter 3, and now it's time to do some hands-on exploration. You can refer to the diagrams in Chapter 3 to remind you of the names of the different parts. You may want privacy for these exercises or you may wish to share the experience with a lover or a partner. Honor whatever needs you have around this. It may be preferable to do this exercise in your bedroom, but you can also do it in the bathroom or anywhere in the house you feel comfortable.

Discovering Your Vulva

This may be the first time you have ever looked closely at your vulva. If so, be prepared to be amazed. Your vulva is the source of tremendous pleasure, and that makes it a thing of beauty. Regardless of how your vulva appears to you now, you can eventually learn to see it as a beautiful flower, an exotic orchid. You may have already looked closely at your vulva and know it well by sight but not be able to identify the different parts. If so, this is your opportunity to discover more.

For this exercise, you will need a handheld mirror and some good lighting. You may want to shower or bathe first and wash your vulva so that she is more presentable for this encounter. You will, of course, need to remove any clothes from the waist down. Find a comfortable seated position with both knees up and splayed apart. If you are in your bed, you can prop yourself up with some pillows behind your back. Then prop the mirror on the bed facing your vulva, freeing both of your hands for exploration. If you need to, you can use one hand for the mirror.

Begin by separating your outer labia with one hand. This will expose your inner labia and your clitoris. Appreciate the delicate tissue there. In your mind, connect how it looks with the exquisite pleasure it is capable of providing you. Notice the flap of tissue at the very top of your inner labia. That is your clitoral hood. You may notice the glans or head of your clitoris poking out from underneath it. Or you may need to pull the hood back a bit, up toward your pubic mound in order to see your clitoris. Touch yourself lightly on top of the clitoral hood first to assess its sensitivity. Then touch the head of your clitoris directly. Touching the head directly should feel considerably more sensitive. Now lightly touch your inner and outer labia to assess the sensitivity of these tissues.

 Essential

Remember, no two vulvas are alike, and there is no right or wrong way for yours to look. Try to regard your vulva with a sense of mystery and curiosity. Notice any judgments you may have about the appearance or your vulva, and then try to just let them go.

After you have seen and touched the different parts of your vulva, spread your inner labia to expose the vestibule. The vestibule consists of your vaginal opening, your Bartholin's glands, and your urethral opening. Gently touch these different parts and notice how they respond to your touch. The location of your vaginal opening should be pretty obvious. It is at the base of the vestibule and will have a puckered appearance. The Bartholin's glands are probably not visible, but by looking at the diagram, you can get a sense of where they are located. Although it is very small, you should be able to see your urethral opening, directly above your vaginal opening. It is a tiny hole. Lightly touch these different parts to get a feel for their sensitivity.

For further discovery, try viewing the inside of your vagina with a speculum. A speculum is a medical instrument that inserts into the vagina and opens enough to allow you to view your vaginal walls and cervix. If you are comfortable with your gynecologist, ask her to show you how to use a speculum, or have her assist you. You can also ask your gynecologist if she has an inexpensive plastic speculum you can take home with you. If you use a speculum at home you will also need a mirror and a flashlight for this exploration.

Discovering Your Penis and Testicles

Being a man, you have probably looked at and touched your penis and testicles plenty, but you may not have studied all the different parts or their names carefully. Also, you may have never assessed the sensitivity of the different parts. This exercise may allow you to get some new information about your penis's and testicles' sensitivity and responsiveness. Start this exercise when your penis is flaccid. If it becomes erect while doing the exercise, that's okay. It is good to notice the differences in sensation between your flaccid penis and your erect penis.

 Alert

It is normal for an erect penis to bend slightly in any which direction and to have some curve in it. If, however, the bending or curving appears suddenly and is accompanied with any swelling or pain, you should consult with a physician.

Start by lightly cupping the scrotal sac that holds your testicles. Notice if one testicle hangs lower than the other, as it does in most men. Notice if one testicle is more sensitive than the other. Notice how your testicles respond to the light cupping. Then, let your hand lightly grip the shaft of your penis, and notice the texture, quality and sensitivity of the skin there. If you are circumcised, lightly touch the exposed glans of your penis. Notice its sensitivity. If you are uncircumcised, pull your foreskin back, exposing the glans, and notice the skin underneath. Touch it lightly, assessing its sensitivity. Then touch the glans itself. Locate the ridged band, the ring of smooth muscle, wrapping around the base of your glans. Softly touch your frenulum, the indentation on the underside of your penis where the glans and the shaft meet. Keep your touch very light, passing a single finger along the ridge and over the frenulum and notice their sensitivity.

Getting to Know Your Erogenous Zones

Your erogenous zones are areas on your body that elicit sexual feelings or sensations. It is possible for your entire body to be an erogenous zone. But for most people, there are just a few specific areas that when touched bring sexual arousal to their bodies. The most obvious and common areas are your genitals. Usually, however, when people refer to erogenous zones, they are referring to other less obvious parts of their bodies that respond erotically when touched.

Possible Erogenous Zones

Erogenous zones tend to be areas on your body that have a lot of nerve endings, or areas where the nerve endings are closest to the surface of the skin, and therefore more accessible. The high density of nerves in certain areas simply means more possibility for stimulation that can make its way to the brain and send out more actions and impulses to the rest of your body. More nerves equal more stimulation. More stimulation equals more arousal and excitement.

Aside from the obvious erogenous zones—the penis, the testicles, the clitoris, the labia, and the vagina—here is a list of other common erogenous zones:

- ears
- feet and toes
- groin
- hands and fingers
- inside of the thighs

- lips, tongue, and mouth
- neck
- perineum
- pubic mound
- sacrum
- scalp
- shoulders
- small of the back
- spine
- stomach
- thighs
- underarms
- underside of the elbows, forearms, and wrists

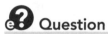 **Question**

What do you need to do to find out where your erogenous zones are?
Discovering your erogenous zones takes some exploration. Make it a priority and set aside some time. You have to be open-minded, interested, curious, patient, and maybe even a little adventuresome. If you are willing to explore, you will reap the rewards in erotic pleasure and bliss, not to mention more interesting and profound orgasms.

Discovering Your Erogenous Zones

What are your erogenous zones? The answer to this question varies from person to person, and your erogenous zones may even vary depending on the situation. For instance, you may need certain erogenous zones stimulated first before others become activated. Direct mental focus or specific kinds of touch are often required to activate an erogenous zone. Light caressing works well for some areas. Others respond better to deeper massaging or squeezing. Some like pinching. Some like to be nibbled on or bit. Some like to be licked or sucked. Some like to be slapped, flogged, or whipped. And still others like to be gently breathed or blown on. Alternatively, sometimes the kind of touch is less important than who is doing the touching.

Body Map Exercise

The body map exercise is a great way to chart your erogenous zones. It involves drawing an outline of your whole body, front and back, on a large piece of paper and then marking your erogenous zones along with descriptions of how those areas like to be stimulated. You will need a big roll of paper, often called butcher paper, at least three feet wide. You can usually find these rolls at art supply stores. You will also need some masking tape, a hard surface, colored markers, and maybe a friend to help.

Cut a piece that is about one and a half feet longer than your body. Tape the paper to a hard floor surface. Lie down on your back, arms slightly away from your body, and legs slightly spread, leaving approximately six inches of paper above your head. Then have a friend, partner, or lover trace the outline of your body using one of the markers. Make sure to spread your fingers and outline all fingers.

 Essential

Save the feet for last, because you will need to cheat in order to draw them, by standing up after the rest of your body is traced and then outlining your feet from a standing position. Again, have your friend trace each toe, by going in between them.

On your body chart, mark your erogenous zones with some marking or symbol that is meaningful to you. Write notes about the kind of touch or stimulation a particular area likes. Use different colors to specify the varying degrees of erotic potential for the different erogenous zones or kinds of touch or stimulation. For example, use purple to mark your nipples as highly erotic zones, or write in red that having your neck gently kissed really turns you on. Then use a different color to mark more subtle erogenous zones and the kinds of stimulation they like. Let yourself be creative.

A really fun way to make your chart is to have a partner help you experiment. Ask him to touch you in various spots with different qualities of touch. What you both learn may make your sex play more enjoyable. Be sure to map your backside on a second sheet of paper.

Connecting the Zones

Your brain is capable of making connections between erogenous zones, and you can enhance this potential with a little practice. Making erogenous zone connections is a concept championed by erotic pioneers Steve and Vera Bodansky, authors of *Instant Orgasm*. They train people to connect the arousal in their genitals to different parts of their bodies. Start by focusing on the arousal in your genitals. Then shift your attention to another part of your body. You can do this cognitively or with the help of touch. Your brain then begins to make associations between the new parts and your overall sexual arousal. You begin to open the channels and enhance the arousal potential of your more subtle erogenous zones. With enough practice, touching the various nongenital parts will signal arousal to your genitals, spreading your potential for pleasure throughout your body. Nifty trick!

 Fact

The term *erogenous zone* was coined at the end of the nineteenth century. It became popularized in the early twentieth century by psychologists who used it to describe how pressure, when applied to certain areas on the body, was capable of generating an orgasm in what were then defined as *hysterical persons*.

Arousal Flow Chart Exercise

The Body Map helps you diagram the areas of your body that give you erotic pleasure, and what kind of stimulation they like. The Arousal Flow Chart, on the other hand, helps you diagram a sequence of erotic stimulation that you either know or suspect could lead you to orgasm.

You may need to do some experimentation to make your arousal flow chart. The first step is to see what gets you started. Play around with the different types of stimulation on different areas of your body. Notice the areas that give you the most amount of erotic charge initially. You may discover that touching or rubbing your genitals really gets things going for you, or you may discover that light caressing all over your body helps you start to build an erotic charge. If you don't already know what has the potential to take you there, experiment and make mental notes about what order of stimulus seems to make you respond the most. Then write down a sequence that you believe would be pleasurable to you.

Here is an example of an arousal flow chart for a woman:

- Lightly caress the front of whole body for five minutes.
- Focus light caresses on belly, sides of body, chest and breasts, avoiding nipples for five minutes.
- Lightly caress face, ears, and neck for three minutes.
- Caress thighs, focusing on inner thighs and groin crease, avoiding genitals for five minutes.
- Caress whole body, focusing most on sides of body, breasts and nipples, neck, inner thighs, and groin crease for ten minutes.
- Focus caressing on inner thighs and groin crease, beginning to tease genitals lightly for five minutes.
- One hand applies lubrication to genitals using very gentle upward strokes, starting from the vaginal opening, across labia, up to clitoris. The other hand moves to stroking breasts and begins to squeeze and pinch nipples for five minutes.

- Begin making light circles and figure-eight motions across clitoris with a pointer finger, mixed in with slow sensual strokes up and down the sides of the inner labia, occasionally dipping fingers lightly into vaginal opening. With the other hand, focus more on nipples, add lubrication, encircle them with one finger, and pinch them for ten minutes.
- Gradually increase frequency and pressure of strokes to vulva, begin dipping fingers more deeply into vagina. Start rocking the pelvis. The other hand continues to play with the nipples for ten minutes.
- One hand now focuses completely on vaginal penetration, stimulating the G-spot with a thrusting action. The other hand alternates between clitoral stimulation and nipple stimulation-until orgasm!

There are endless possibilities for arousal flow charts. Each person may have her own unique version. Or you may have several different versions that all work well. If you have a sequence you know satisfies you, consider adding some creative variations. Variety can spice things up and prevent you from falling into a routine that loses excitement over time.

CHAPTER 5

Practicing Alone
or Playing Solo

Pleasuring your body by yourself has two primary and exciting benefits. One is learning how to play your instrument better, without the pressure of performing in front of others. The other is the sheer enjoyment of the pleasure you can create for yourself. Whenever you are tired of delayed gratification, consider giving yourself whatever you want, right now. Every musician knows the value of practicing her instrument alone and the joy of playing solo.

Self-Pleasuring

Self-pleasuring is the art of giving oneself sensual and erotic pleasure. It is used here in place of its synonym, masturbation. For many people, the term *masturbation* has a negative connotation, since it has long been a highly stigmatized activity in many cultures. For others, the term masturbation sounds too clinical. It may sound like something you do to merely release sexual tension. The term self-pleasuring, on the other hand, is broader, implying sensual as well as sexual enjoyment. Many people have come up with their own, often humorous, idioms for masturbation, from "spanking the monkey" or "choking the chicken" to "airing the orchid" or "teasing the kitty." You may have your own unique expression for it. No matter what you call it, it is your birthright and there are many benefits to making it a practice in your life.

Self-Loving Pioneers

In the 1950s, Alfred Kinsey's studies on human sexual behavior showed that masturbation was a normal sexual behavior that most men and many women participate in regularly. Subsequent pioneers such as Lonnie Barbach, Betty Dodson, and Joseph Kramer have helped take masturbation, self-loving, and orgasms to a whole new level through books, videos, workshops, and individual coaching. Their work has been crucial in bringing sexual awareness and healing to the forefront of today's culture.

Why Self-Pleasure?

To some, the answer to this question may seem obvious, but there are actually many reasons that people self-pleasure. It is a worthwhile activity not only for the sake of achieving orgasm, although that may be the most common reason. The following are just a few of the reasons you may choose to engage in the act of self-pleasuring.

- Perhaps for you, self-pleasuring is a way to relieve sexual tension. You may feel a sexual tension building inside you that needs periodic release. This may be simply a byproduct of your body's natural sex drive. Accumulated sexual tension might also be a result of exposure to something you find sexually stimulating, an image or an interaction with someone who turns you on. Self-pleasuring for this reason is about following an internal impulse.
- You may not experience the build-up of erotic energy on its own, but you may want to feel more sexual pleasure in your body. You may self-pleasure as a way to build arousal and enjoy more pleasurable erotic sensations. In this case, you

may or may not choose to complete your self-pleasuring with an orgasm.

- You may self-pleasure as a way to help you relax or sleep better. Orgasm can have a highly sedative effect on the body. It is often used as a sleep aid. It is much healthier than using pharmaceutical medications and much more enjoyable than counting sheep.

- Self-pleasuring can help you learn about your sexuality. It's a great way to experiment and figure out what works for you. If you have difficulty with early ejaculation, you can work on prolonging arousal through masturbation. If you have difficulty with orgasm, you can experiment with different sequences and intensities of stimulation, or with different fantasy scenarios. Self-pleasuring can help you discover what your sexual needs are so that you can communicate those needs in sexual encounters with others.

- Self-pleasuring offers you autonomy over your sexuality. You are less dependent upon others when you know you can take matters into your own hands. Self-pleasuring allows you to stay sexually active when you don't have a lover or when your lover is unavailable. If you have a lover who has a less frequent interest in sex than you, masturbation can help reduce potential power struggles over how often you have sex.

- Finally, self-pleasuring can give you energy, make you feel sexy and beautiful, and make you appreciate and love your body more. It can be a way to honor and love and worship yourself, body and soul.

Masturbation Guilt

Many people feel guilty when they masturbate. This unfortunate phenomenon is usually the result of the sex-negative messages espoused by religious or other cultural influences. Serious masturbation guilt sometimes has devastating psychological consequences, including suicide. In particular, young men with strong natural biological urges may become distraught and psychologically conflicted if they are taught that masturbation is shameful.

 Essential

The Biblical story of Onan is often cited as proof that masturbation is a sin. Onan was supposed to impregnate his dead brother's wife, as was the law in those times. He chose, however, to "spill his seed" instead. This was considered evil, and therefore God took Onan's life.

Bad for Your Health?

There are many myths about masturbation being bad for your health. In the Victorian era, the medical profession joined forces with the moralists of the day, condemning masturbation as an activity to be feared. It was believed to be detrimental to one's physical and mental health, capable of causing a plethora of problems in the young and old. A variety of methods, many of which were quite absurd and even torturous, were invented at this time to prevent children and adults from masturbating. No wonder people today still have a hard time admitting that they masturbate!

In ancient times, it was believed that a man had only a limited supply of sperm. This sperm was considered to contain a man's life force. Therefore, masturbation was thought to deplete his life force and was therefore not considered to be a healthy activity. Even today, some Taoist practices that are becoming popular in the West train men to orgasm without ejaculation, so as not to deplete their life force. While there is nothing wrong with learning this practice, there is no medical evidence that semen contains a man's life force. Even though modern science and medicine know better, there are still people who believe masturbation to be harmful to their health.

Good for Your Health!

Contrary to the myths, modern science and medicine find that masturbation is actually good for your health for many reasons. For starters, masturbation is the safest sex you can have. You need not worry about catching any colds or diseases from yourself. Self-pleasuring helps relieve tension and stress in the whole body. This can positively affect the immune system. Masturbation can help to alleviate menstrual cramps in women. It can take away headaches and it helps keep the muscles of the pelvic floor toned, which can help prevent urinary incontinence as you age. All these benefits come with no proven negative side effects.

 Fact

A recent medical study concluded that frequent masturbation actually reduces the risk of prostate cancer in men. This is because cancer-causing chemicals may build up in the prostate when men do not ejaculate on a regular basis. Intercourse, however, does not have the same protective effect, due to the chances of contracting a sexually transmitted disease, which increases men's cancer risk.

The Basics of Getting Down with Yourself

There is no right or wrong way to get it on with yourself. Remember, you are your own authority when it comes to your sexuality! Where you do it, why you do it, and how you do it, is all up to you and you alone. Let yourself try new things. When you are alone, no one can judge you or hold you back, so play, explore, and have fun with yourself!

The Venue

Where you choose to make your own sweet music is up to you. First of all, there is nothing that says you need to be lying in a bed while self-pleasuring. This is often the safest and most comfortable place people think of to masturbate or have sex, but it is not necessarily the most erotic or exciting. Don't limit yourself! You are free to self-pleasure wherever you feel comfortable and safe and are not likely to offend anyone. So try different places: your kitchen or bathroom, a hallway, or somewhere out in nature, if you are sure you won't be seen.

Visual Stimulation

Many people enjoy some visual stimulation during the act of self-pleasuring. Viewing erotic images can help spark up your arousal level. Men are known for using erotic magazines or videos more for this purpose, but many women also indulge in erotic imagery to help with arousal. Unfortunately, some aspects of pornography may turn you off as much as others turn you on. If so, choose a media that works well for you and leave the rest behind. Whether you use mental imagery, fantasy, erotica, or pornography, you should not feel ashamed. Images of people being sexual are naturally arousing.

Self-Touch

Touching yourself well is perhaps the greatest gift you can give yourself. It is a gesture of self-love that will help create a positive feedback loop for your body and mind. Offer your body the attention it deserves and it will offer you more pleasure. In addition, the more you touch yourself, the more you learn what touch feels good to you, and the more you can tell your lover what you like.

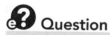 **Question**

What kind of touch is erotically stimulating?
Different kinds of touch work at different times on different parts of your body. Feather-light stroking with your fingertips, full-hand caressing, kneading, pinching, squeezing, tapping and slapping, pounding, pressing, and pulsing or vibrating are some of the things you can try to different parts of your body. See what works for you!

Becoming Orgasmic

Reaching orgasm is a real challenge for some people. In general, women tend to struggle with this more often than men. If you are pre-orgasmic (have not yet experienced orgasm) or just find that you are challenged in this area, then self-pleasuring may be your key to unlocking the mystery. Spend a lot of time with the exercises in this chapter. It may take two hours or more of self-caressing, direct stimulation, and fantasy exploration to discover your full sexual response. The trick is persistence, an open mind, and a willingness to be creative while staying focused on pleasurable sensations in your body. Unless there is a medical reason preventing it, you can orgasm if you give it enough time and attention.

Become a Connoisseur of Your Own Pleasure

Self-pleasuring has the potential to be much more than just getting off. There is a time and place for the simple and quick release of sexual tension. Sometimes, however, you might choose to go for more than that. Why not give yourself the gift of an erotic ride that will nourish you, inspire you, and make you feel more alive? Self-pleasuring is an art, a great art. And you are the artist capable of creating your own ecstatic collage of feelings and sensations.

Developing Your Technique

You may have already figured out a way to masturbate that brings you significant arousal and helps you achieve orgasm. However, there are undoubtedly things that you have not yet considered or tried. The following suggestions for stimulating your genitals can help you add to an expanding repertoire.

Stimulating Your Vulva

Begin by spending a fair amount of time warming yourself up before starting in on your vulva. Caress and tease your whole body before you zero in on your genitals. When you are ready, begin by making sure your vulva is nicely lubed up. Depending on your body and the time of month, you may already have enough natural lubrication to play with. If you feel a little dry (which is normal), that is easily remedied. Your own saliva is readily available and has a great consistency for sliding and gliding your fingers around your vulva. However, if you prefer, try some oil or commercial personal lubricants. There are many options; Chapter 12 discusses sexual lubricants in more detail.

Caressing and Massaging the Vulva

Begin by putting your own saliva, some oil, or personal lube onto the fingertips of the hand you will be using to stimulate your vulva. Apply the lubrication in gentle strokes, starting at your vaginal opening and moving upward, dragging your fingers slowly across and on either side of your inner labia, ending with the tip of your middle finger on your clitoris. Repeat this, moving your fingers slightly until your entire vulva is well lubricated, or as long as it continues to feel pleasurable. Allow your fingers and your whole hand to remain relaxed. Pause briefly between each stroke.

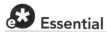 **Essential**

Throughout your self-pleasuring session, continue to focus on the pleasurable sensations in your vulva and the rest of your body. Relax your body and deepen your breath. Anticipate each stroke before you place your hand on your vulva to begin again. This will help you build more arousal.

Once your vulva is nicely lubed, you may be ready to try some new strokes. Continue exploring the different parts of your vulva with varying amounts of pressure and speed. Focus on the pleasurable sensations and let them guide you. What increases the pleasure at any given moment: A lighter touch or firmer pressure? Try speeding the strokes up or slowing them down—alternate between fast and slow. Do you like little circles or long strokes? Try letting your fingers engage in a dance of chaos. See if you can surprise yourself. Play with intermittingly pinching, squeezing, and pulling your clitoris and labia. Keep applying lubrication as needed to keep it juicy.

Stimulating the Clitoris

Your clitoris may or may not want direct stimulation. The clitoris has more nerve endings per square inch than any other part of your body, making it extremely sensitive to touch. You may only want to touch your clitoris over the clitoral hood or possibly stay away from it altogether. Or you may find that your clitoris may enjoy vigorous touch. The clitoris will still receive some stimulation regardless of whether or not you touch it directly. When you become aroused and the blood starts to flow into the erectile tissue, your clitoris will also become engorged and stimulated.

If you like the sensation of touching your clitoris, try pinching it between two fingers, and gliding the hood back and forth over it. You can also try pulling the hood back, up toward the pubis mons, with two fingers of one hand. Then use the tip of a finger on the other hand to gently stimulate the head of your clitoris directly. Try a lateral stroke, side-to-side, crossing over the clitoris, while applying varying degrees of pressure. Circles and figure eights over the clitoris can also feel incredibly good. Notice if one side of your clitoris is more sensitive than another. A gentle upward stroke with a fingertip on the more sensitive side may be very pleasurable.

 Fact

Some research has shown that the upper left quadrant of the clitoral head in many women is the most sensitive spot and the most responsive to pleasurable sensations. Of course, there are no universal truths when it comes to this kind of statement, but it is well worth checking out for yourself!

Involving Your Erogenous Zones

Your other hand has many options for getting in on the action. It can continue to caress and stroke different parts of your body and erogenous zones. Your lips, mouth, face, ears, and neck may want some attention. Or perhaps your breasts and nipples are yearning to be caressed, squeezed, or pinched. Try lightly stroking your inner thighs. Or maybe it's all hands on deck, i.e. both hands focusing on the genitals. Your second hand can help by pressing on your mons pubis, pulling back the hood of your clitoris, separating your labia, or penetrating your vagina or anus. Allow your second hand to roam and continue to freely explore the options.

Use That PC Muscle

Self-pleasuring is the perfect time to practice squeezing your love muscle (see the pelvic floor exercise in Chapter 2). Your heightened awareness of your vulva at this time may also help you differentiate your PC muscle from the other pelvic floor muscles. Try spending a considerable amount of time just squeezing and relaxing your PC muscle. This should stimulate your vulva and help direct more blood into the tissues there. See if that increases your pleasure or arousal. Try combining this with some fantasy and see how close you can come to climax without ever touching yourself.

Move Your Body

Let your whole body be involved in self-pleasuring. There's no reason you should stay in one position or remain still the whole time. Try different positions. Get up on all fours—doggie-style—and see how you like that. Try standing up, or leaning against a wall. Try bending over a desk or table. Get creative with positioning your body and see how the different positions stimulate your fantasies. Alternatively, let your fantasies inspire different body positions. You may want to move your body while self-pleasuring. Your pelvis may want to rock. Try pushing with your legs to gently rock your entire body. See how different movements contribute to your arousal.

Make Noise

Making noise and continuing to breathe deeply into your belly can really increase pleasure in your whole body. Let yourself sigh and moan and groan or squeal and scream in whatever way you are moved. Making noises can instigate a positive feedback loop. You make a noise that expresses your arousal level and the noise itself may arouse you even more. Breathing deeply into your belly will keep your attention on your body and keep your blood well-oxygenated.

Try a Sex Toy

If you would like to give your hand a break or if you find you need more stimulation than your hand can provide, you can try using a vibrator. Many women experience their first orgasm with the aid of a vibrator. The sensations can be very intense at first. Be sure to start the vibrator on a low setting and avoid putting it directly on your clitoris. You can either stimulate the tissue around your clitoris, your groin and/or your labia, or you can put a towel or some heavy material between the vibrator and your vulva.

 Alert

You can over-stimulate the nerves in the clitoris and make it so that they become a bit desensitized to more subtle stimulation. Give your body a chance to respond to a lighter stimulus first. If you have tried many times and just know your body needs a vibrator to become aroused or reach orgasm, then by all means, fire it up!

If you would like to play more with penetration of your vagina or anus during your self-pleasuring, you can enlist the aid of dildos or butt plugs. In a pinch, many women have experimented with various fruits and vegetables (bananas and cucumbers work well) or household objects such as hairbrush handles or pencils. This is up to you and your imagination. More information on using vibrators, dildos, and other sex toys is available in Chapter 12.

Stimulating Your Penis

Most men have some, if not a lot, of familiarity with masturbation. Self-pleasuring in a more global sense, however, may be a new idea. To experiment, take some time, deliberately not touching your penis at first. Instead, let your hands caress your whole body, the same way a lover's hands would caress you if you were with a partner. In fact, imagine yourself as your own lover. Touch yourself with the same sense of erotic mystique you would touch someone you desired. Find your erogenous zones and give them the attention they deserve, releasing the pleasure they have to offer.

Once you have spent a good amount of time stimulating and awakening your whole body through self-touch and caressing, you can move on to touching, squeezing, caressing, and stroking your penis.

 Essential

In general, stroking your penis feels best when you use lubrication. Find lubrication that works for you. For some, this will be your own sweet saliva. Others may want to use oil or a commercial personal lubricant. Apply liberally and frequently to keep it juicy.

Begin by placing some lube on the tips of your middle and index fingers and thumb of the hand you will be using on your penis. Start out with very gentle strokes from the head of the penis down to the base. When you get to the base of your penis, remove your hand and begin the stroke again from the head of your penis on down rather than stroking back upward. Continue in this manner, moving your fingers slightly with each stroke, until your whole penis is covered with lube, or as long as this keeps feeling good.

When you are ready for more stimulation, you may add more lube to your hand and begin to use your whole hand. Try continuing to stroke your penis only in downward movements, lifting your hand each time you reach the base. Pause between each stroke and bring your awareness to the pleasurable sensations there. Breathe deeply. Anticipate the next stroke before you put your hand on your penis to continue stroking. Enjoy the pleasurable sensations of the anticipation. This will let the energy continue to build slowly and help you bring more of your focus onto the pleasure, rather than the task at hand. It can also help you increase your ability to contain more of an erotic charge in your body without automatically amplifying or releasing it.

Once you have explored slow, deliberate stroking to your satisfaction, let go and follow the flow of sexual energy you feel. Allow your hand to move up and down your penis in whatever way it is called to do. Tap into the pleasure of your body and let it guide you. Allow yourself to continue to use fantasy or visual stimulation freely, especially if it helps you heighten your arousal.

 Alert

> While masturbating is a healthy activity, masturbation habits that interfere or endanger your reputation or other goals in your life could be a sign of sex addiction. If you find you are masturbating in ways that feel unhealthy and out of your control, then you should seek professional help.

A Sacred Solo Ritual

To further your adventures in self-pleasure, consider making love to yourself in the context of a sacred solo ritual. It can be very liberating and expansive to regard masturbation as something that is worthy of the respect inherent in the practice of ritual. This can turn the tables on any shame you might feel.

Give yourself at least two hours for this ritual. This is an opportunity to bring the power of your self-loving into a context that can provide a tremendous amount of nourishment for your body-mind connection and your soul. Because you are taking your time to get into your pleasure body and build arousal, this ritual also has the capacity to provide you with incredibly rich, satisfying, and meaningful orgasms, worthy of a standing ovation were anyone to be witnessing them! This can become a weekly or a monthly ritual, something you do just for yourself to increase your own self-nurturance, rejuvenate yourself, and stoke your life force fires.

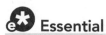 **Essential**

Be sure to create a safely contained environment for this ritual. Turn off the ringer on the phone. Put a "Do not Disturb" sign on the door, if needed. Arrange for any children or pets to be cared for so that they will not be a distraction or a nuisance.

Create Sacred Space

Set the stage for your ritual by creating a beautiful and comfortable environment in which you feel nourished, warm, safe, and relaxed. Heat the space if it is cold. Light some candles. Lay down a soft blanket or beautiful tapestry on the bed or the floor where you will be making love to yourself. Throw some soft pillows down to both beautify the space and create more comfort. You may want to burn some sage or incense or use an aromatherapy diffuser to flavor the air with a pleasant scent. Put some nice soothing music on to caress your eardrums and touch your soul.

Bathe or Shower

Next, treat yourself to a long hot bath or shower. If you like, use scented soap, shower gel, or bubble bath to delight your olfactory system. While in the shower or bath, let yourself begin to relax.

Really take in the pleasurable sensation of warmth on your skin. Immerse your whole body, including your hair and face, in the water. Delight in the wetness.

If you are taking a shower, let the water hit your tongue and enter your mouth. Enjoy the feeling of warm water raining down on your face and neck. Turn around slowly and savor the feeling of the hot water pounding on your shoulders and back. If you are taking a bath, take a deep breath and immerse yourself completely, allowing your neck and head to release any tension. Let your body just float effortlessly. When you apply the soap or shower gel, take your time and enjoy slow sensual caresses. Stay in the bath or shower as long as you like, but make sure it is at least twenty minutes.

Dress for the Occasion

Now it is time to dress yourself in something that is comfortable and makes you look and feel fabulous and sexy. This could be any number of outfits: lingerie, underwear, leather pants, a summer dress, a sarong, or just your birthday suit. Use your imagination. Wear whatever you think will make this ritual special to you and help you feel attractive.

Honor Your Image

The next part of the ritual involves spending some time in front of a full-length mirror. This is a time to visually appreciate your image. Notice what you like about your looks and affirm your appreciation out loud. For example, if you like the color of your hair, you might say, "I like the deep chestnut color of my hair, and I think it is beautiful." Focus only on what you like and feel good about. Be as detailed and specific as you can. Find at least five things to appreciate about your appearance.

Honor Yourself

Next, enter the space you created at the beginning of the ritual. Sit or kneel on the blanket or tapestry. Take a moment to appreciate yourself for setting aside this time and making your self-pleasure a priority. You may want to make a gesture with this appreciation, putting your hands on your heart or in a prayer position. If it works for you, bow your head and take a deep breath. You may also take this opportunity to acknowledge the awesomeness of your existence and your gratitude for a body capable of so much pleasure.

 Fact

Some ancient cultures revered masturbation as a symbol of renewal. It was thought of as a way to unleash pent-up emotions, unlock the flow of the body's energy, and reconnect with nature. In Egyptian mythology, the Egyptian god Atum rose from the chaos to create the air, the moisture, the earth, and the sky through the act of masturbation.

Caress Yourself

Lie down in a comfortable position, propped up with pillows where necessary, and continue loving and appreciating yourself while caressing your whole body. You may use your hands or you may choose to use a feather or feather duster. Notice any negative thoughts, criticisms, or judgments that come up, and do as much as you can to just let them go. Keep focusing your mind on appreciative thoughts and gratitude. Cultivating positive, self-loving thoughts is a practice that requires some discipline. Eventually, the loving self-touch you give yourself and the positive thoughts your mind generates will create a positive feedback loop, and the two will flow seamlessly together without any effort.

Tease Yourself

While you touch yourself, let your genitals be a focal point around which you touch without giving them direct attention initially. This will help build up an erotic charge, and may be more effective than actually touching your genitals directly. Teasing yourself increases the tension by heightening your sense of

The Everything Orgasm Book

anticipation. With a light touch, work all around your inner thighs, in the creases of your groin, on your buttocks, and in your butt crack. Stimulate your anus and perineum. Gently stroke and tug on your pubic hair. If you are a man, tickle your testicles. Feel the urge to be touched on your genitals building and increasing in intensity. But hold off for a while. See how much erotic charge you can build this way.

Stimulate Your Genitals

Begin this portion of the ritual with one hand on your heart and the other on your genitals. Rest there for a few minutes, breathing in the sensations and allowing a connection to be made between your heart and genitals. Here you can affirm your love for your erotic body and appreciation for all the sexual pleasure your body is capable of. Follow the suggestions from the previous section on techniques for stimulating your vulva or your penis. Continue to weave in affirmations of self-love and appreciation.

Ending the Ritual

There is no clear end to this ritual. You may decide that you arc done in two hours. You may decide that you are done once you have had an orgasm. You may end when you feel emotionally full and satisfied. It is up to you. When you do feel complete, take a moment once again to honor yourself for giving yourself this sacred time. You may once again gesture with your hands over your heart and bow, if that feels appropriate. Acknowledge yourself for the vital life force that you are, the good you are capable of, and the pleasure that is your birthright.

CHAPTER 6

Harmonizing
with Your Lover

The pleasure our bodies can feel is a great gift. Combine that gift with a sense of connection to someone you care about and you can open yourself to even greater satisfaction. Having a lover to play with creates many new options for enjoying your sexuality. But it can also invite more complexity and complications. It helps to attend to your relationship and keep your relationship in harmony, making sure you both get what you need.

Loving Yourself

The best thing you can offer a partner is a good, solid relationship with yourself.

Centering and Grounding

Centering and grounding is the process of regaining balance and solidity in yourself. Some people center themselves by reminding themselves of their inherent worthiness and lovability. Others may recall their spiritual connection to something greater than themselves. When you are centered and grounded, you know where you stand in relation to the world around you. You are not easily unnerved or agitated. You can show up in a way that allows you be fully present with others.

Tracking Your Own Needs

Loving yourself also involves taking care of yourself and your needs and desires. Humans are a very social species. We all need connection, love and respect. We also need autonomy, freedom and acceptance. Unfortunately, most people have been shamed for having these essential human needs. And sexual needs and desires are often shamed the most.

Satisfying your sexual needs starts with acknowledging and accepting them. Once you've done this, you have to take charge to make sure you get what you need. You can meet some needs on your own, but you can engage others to help you meet other needs. Ultimately, you alone are responsible for making sure your needs are met. There is no better person for the job. Nobody could possibly track your needs as well as you.

Your ability to insure your own satisfaction relieves others of this burden. One of the greatest pleasures of partner-sex is enjoying how much pleasure you can offer someone else. When you can make sure you get what you need, you are helping your partner be successful at satisfying you. Sex is a game where everyone can win, but only if you both make sure you get what you need.

Finding Your Voice

Successfully getting what you need usually requires being able to express your desires and preferences. Once you are clear about what you want, you have to be able to convey it to your partner. Expecting your partner to read your mind doesn't work. The ability to communicate will both increase your satisfaction and make you a better lover. No sexual technique or chemistry can replace communication about what you or your partner need in each moment. Sex is a time to speak up.

Talking about Sex

Being comfortable talking about sex is a rare skill. It is generally not learned in school or in the home. Sex is such a taboo subject that it may be hard to push through the thick cloak of shame or awkwardness surrounding it. Not communicating about sex, however, can put both your health and your enjoyment at risk. Here are some things you need to be able to talk about to have healthy, safe, and enjoyable sex.

Safe Sex Talk

Before you begin to be sexual with a new lover, make sure you talk about your recent sexual history and any precautions that may be needed to keep sex between you safe. This will enable you to make good decisions about how you proceed sexually. It is important that both partners understand how sexual diseases are transmitted and how transmission can be prevented. It is also important to assess the degree of risk that either of you may unknowingly have a sexually transmitted disease (STD). Here are some of the topics covered in a good safe sex discussion:

- Do you have any STDs that you are aware of?
- Have you recently been tested for STDs?
- Which infections were you tested for and when?
- What sexual activity have you had since your last testing?
- Were bodily fluids exchanged in that activity?
- What protections do you want to employ in sex with this partner?
- What sexual activities do you want to rule out, for safety's sake?

Always keep in mind that ensuring your sexual health is your own responsibility. Even covering these topics will not ensure that your partner has been completely open or accurate in his or her responses. The risks are particularly high with new sexual partners, with whom you may not have had time to develop trust. If you want to stay healthy, make sure you are fully informed about the most current information on safe sex and that you always protect yourself.

 Fact

Sexually transmitted diseases (STDs) are infectious diseases transmitted through the exchange of bodily fluids—semen, blood, saliva—during vaginal, oral, or anal sexual activity. It is possible to have an STD and have no symptoms. You or your lover could be unaware that you have an infection.

Satisfying Preconditions

Everyone has preconditions for sex. Your preconditions are the conditions you need to have in place before you can be fully open to a sexual interaction. They include things like being with the right person, being in an appropriate relationship, being well-rested, being relaxed, feeling emotionally connected, and having sufficient privacy. Everyone has his own personal set of preconditions. Some people have a short list; they are ready for almost anything, anytime, anywhere, with anyone. Others may have a longer list and need many more conditions to be in place to feel comfortable engaging in a sexual encounter. No one's list is wrong. Your preconditions are simply an honest personal account of what conditions allow you to feel comfortable entering into sexual activity.

Knowing your preconditions for sex and having them satisfied makes sex and orgasms much more satisfying. Thus, letting your partner know about your preconditions can improve your sexual relationship. When you work together to make sure both partners' preconditions are met, then sex can proceed easily. Communication about preconditions can help you avoid the power struggle that often develops when one person is ready for sex and the other is not.

Saying What You Want

In order for you to have your sexual wishes fulfilled, you will need to be able to say what you want. This requires knowing what you want and having the confidence to ask for it. Sometimes you might not be sure what you want. The self-pleasuring exercises in Chapter 5 are helpful for those who want to learn more about themselves prior to bringing on a partner. But it is also possible to explore the possibilities together. Consider asking your partner to help you explore what feels good. Agree that it is okay to just experiment and learn what each of you likes.

 Alert

Perhaps you know exactly what you want, but you are scared to ask for it. You may be uncertain how your lover will respond to your desires. If this is the case, you may need to share your vulnerable feelings first and request that your partner be sensitive to your feelings around you desires.

Sharing wants and longings can make you feel vulnerable, but it is the way to having them satisfied. Once it is clear that you need your partner to be sensitive to the desires you are about to express, it may be easier to speak them.

Giving and Receiving Feedback

Giving and receiving feedback is an art, and can take a great deal of practice. It is essential to learn this art in order to get the most out of your sexual encounters. In general, it is best when feedback is delivered clearly and sensitively, but not overly so. Complaining, blaming, and shaming never go over well. It works much better to ask clearly for what you do want, rather than telling your partner what she is doing wrong.

One formula for giving feedback is to sandwich what you would like to be different in some way between two things you enjoy how your lover does already. For example, "I really like the pressure you're using on my clitoris right now. Could you slow it down a little bit? That's the perfect amount of lube too." This would probably be better received than: "Whoa! Could you slow it down already! That's way too fast!" It is important to work with your lover to determine how each of you likes to receive feedback and tailor it to your individual needs.

 Essential

When giving feedback, make sure it comes out as a request, not a demand. Your lover doesn't want to feel like he is being ordered around when he is only trying to please you. If you want your lover to keep trying to please you, then be gracious with your feedback.

Receiving feedback can be tricky too. But it is definitely something you want to encourage in your relationship. The more feedback your lover gives you, the better lover you can be for him. Consider thanking your lover for feedback, even when it is negative or poorly delivered. Then adjust or modify what you are doing. Finally, check in with your partner to see if your adjustment improved his experience.

Above all, try not to get defensive. Defensiveness is likely to inhibit your lover from giving you feedback in the future. Ultimately this will undermine your ability to be a good lover. It may even make your partner less interested in sex with you. Remember that it may be difficult for your partner to give feedback, particularly if he is not skilled in the art. He needs your patience and compassion, not your wounded pride.

Sexual Relationship Dynamics

Intimate sexual relationships have the potential to be the most profound and satisfying relationships you can have. They can also be the scariest, most challenging, and most frustrating. Some patterns occur commonly and are worth identifying so you can deal with them better.

Types of Relationships

There are many kinds of sexual relationships, with varying degrees of connection and commitment. Some lovers are in a committed monogamous relationship. Others have varying degrees of involvement other than having sex. Lovers can be partners for just a one-night stand. They can be friends with privileges. Some are in love. Some are not. There are many possibilities. Regardless of the type of relationship you have with a lover, the act of sex can generate some interesting dynamics between two (or more!) people.

Fear of Intimacy

Most people have some degree of fear about intimacy. Perhaps being close to someone brings up concerns about your autonomy. Perhaps closeness triggers past memories of rejection or abandonment. Sometimes sexual intimacy awakens needs for nurturing that went unmet in childhood. Sometimes being sexual will uncover painful past memories of abuse. Intimacy can evoke overwhelming feelings. Successfully dealing with these feelings can stop them from interfering with your enjoyment of sex and orgasm. It can also bring you closer to your partner.

> **EXERCISE:** If you are currently in a relationship, talk with your partner about the feelings that intimacy brings up within you. It is important to share this information so that your partner knows that this is part of the package that is you. If you need support, consulting a therapist can be very helpful.

Sexual Vulnerability

Sex is a vulnerable act. In addition to fears of intimacy, sex can expose shame about your body or anxiety about your performance. It can challenge your ability to communicate well and take care of yourself. It can be scary. Sometimes, sex can hurt. It is important to acknowledge this. People engaging in sex are exposing vulnerabilities to each other. The more trust and sensitivity you can bring to the relationship, the better your lovemaking will go. Leave judgments behind and allow yourselves to feel your feelings, whatever they may be. That will enable you to open to the greatest enjoyment.

Sexual Compatibility

Two partners are most sexually compatible when they have similar arousal maps. When both people like the same activities, there may be an easy flow through the stages of arousal. No two sexualities are exactly the same, however. Your arousal map is inevitably different from your lover's in some regard. For instance, one of you may love kissing and really needs a lot of it to get turned on enough to do anything else. The other may not like kissing at all. If so, you have a challenge to your sexual compatibility.

Sexual compatibility can be enhanced in two ways. First, you can simply take turns pleasuring each other. It can be a real joy to offer your partner exactly what she most wants, even if it is not particularly arousing for you. Both of you can get your needs met if you focus on each other, one at a time. Secondly, you can learn to expand your arousal map. The things that turn your partner on may be things you could open up to enjoying as well. In Chapter 4 you learned that you can enhance enjoyment of your erogenous zones by connecting them to the pleasure of your genitals. Likewise, activities that do not initially excite you may become more arousing as you repeatedly associate them with the excitement your partner feels about them.

Discrepancy in Desire

A discrepancy in desire is a very common phenomenon in relationships wherein one person wants more sexual interaction than the other. Since no two sexualities are the same, this is to be expected. There is no right or wrong amount of desire for sexual connection. There are only different amounts. Dealing with a discrepancy usually requires some compromise from both parties. The partner that wants more sex more often may need to take care of his own needs more by self-pleasuring. The partner less interested in sex at the time may be willing to assist her lover by kissing or stroking him while he self-pleasures. There are many ways to make creative compromises that work for all parties involved.

Couples dealing with significant differences in desire levels can benefit from paying close attention to the preconditions for sex held by the partner with less frequent desire. Working together to meet these preconditions is the most cooperative way to enjoy more satisfaction with sex.

 Alert

Pressuring your lover to have sex when her preconditions are not met is usually counter-productive. It can actually make sex less frequent, because a power struggle prevents authentic sexual desire from freely emerging. Similarly, neglecting to create conditions under which you are likely to feel sexual may also undermine your own enjoyment as well as the health of your relationship.

Making Time for Sex

There is a common belief that sex should be spontaneous. You and your lover may have the kind of lifestyle that allows for that. But if you don't, you may need to actually schedule a regular time for sex if it's going to happen with any consistency. This is particularly true in relationships where the two of you have been together for a while or when there are kids in the picture. There is no reason why sex can't be planned. You plan other enjoyable activities, like going out to eat, going for a walk, and going to the movies. If you know your preconditions for sex, then satisfying them can be a part of getting you in the mood. Of course, if the time comes and it is not possible to meet your preconditions, no one should feel that he has to have sex simply because it says so on the calendar.

Initiating Sex

Another common dynamic in couples is the question of who initiates sex and how they go about it. Sometimes the person who wants sex more often is the one who tends to initiate it. Sometimes, to reduce the incidence of rejected offers, initiation is left up to the person who wants sex less often. Sometimes couples take turns, each enjoying both asking and being asked. You may want to consider how sex is initiated in your relationship and whether you are happy or frustrated with your dynamic.

There are several common frustrations. You may not like how often your initiatives are turned down. You may not like feeling pressured to be sexual when you are not in the mood. You may want to be wooed, wined, and dined. Or you may prefer to be asked directly. You may want to be the seducer some of the time and be seduced at other times.

 Fact

Studies have shown that men tend to initiate sex an average of three times more frequently than women. Studies have also shown that for couples in which initiation of sex is more equal, both women and men are more sexually satisfied. Surprise!

The key to resolving these frustrations is to talk together about your preconditions for sex. If you get rejected often, you can reduce the incidence by putting more energy into satisfying your partner's preconditions and less effort into asking for sex when you know those preconditions are not met. If you feel pressure from your partner, you can take charge of the situation by meeting your own preconditions and expressing more clearly what you do want from your partner.

Intimacy-Enhancing Exercises

For some people, arousal and orgasm come most easily when there is a feeling of emotional closeness with a lover. For others, sex does not require intimacy, but it is enriched when it includes emotional bonding. Intimacy can be either a precondition for sex or a valuable sexual enhancement. Regardless of how long you have been with your lover, and even if it's just an affair, these exercises can help you become a better lover by bringing more intimacy into your relationship.

Hand On Heart

The heart is often the first place in your body where fear shows up. When sharing your feelings with a lover, you may have some vulnerability and fear. It can feel very nurturing and soothing to have your lover's hand over your heart while you share your vulnerable feelings. In this exercise you take turns with your lover sharing your feelings. Give yourselves fifteen to thirty minutes each for this exercise.

The person who is going to share first lies down on a bed or the floor. The other person sits next to him, at about waist level, facing him, and places her dominant hand over his heart. (If you are right handed, your right sides will be next to each other; if you are left-handed, your left sides will be next to each other.) The person who is going to share takes his time to begin. You can take some deep breaths, relax, and feel the warmth and softness of your lover's hand on your heart. When you are ready, speak from your heart about how you are feeling. Try to use "I" statements. Stay away from "you" statements. In other words, express how you are feeling, not what you perceive your lover is doing, thinking, or feeling.

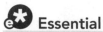

Essential

If you have a fear or concern that your lover has thoughts or feelings that scare you, you can express that fear, but stay away from judgments. Judgments are likely to make your lover defensive, which can create or exacerbate negative thoughts and feelings in your lover.

As the listener, listen with your heart, and stay focused on a feeling of empathy. You are not to fix or change how your lover is feeling. You are just giving him your undivided, loving attention as he shares how he is feeling. If strong feelings begin to emerge, simply breathe deeply and stay in a calm, loving, and nurturing state, allowing whatever waves of emotion to pass through. When your lover is done sharing, thank him for sharing his feelings and allowing you to witness his vulnerability. Take as much time as you need to transition to your time to share.

Eye Gazing

Looking into a lover's eyes without saying anything can be a very scary thing for some people. You may see something you don't want to see, or feel something you don't want to feel. You may be afraid that your lover will see something in you that you don't want him to see. Looking into your lover's eyes and holding her gaze is a way to connect deeply. A lot can be transmitted through the eyes. It is a way to feel more secure, attached, and connected with a lover. In mutual eye gazing you just stay present with whatever emotions come up. It is a chance to explore whatever feelings you have about witnessing and being witnessed by your lover through each other's eyes.

For this exercise, sit in a comfortable position directly across from your lover. Set a timer for five or ten minutes. Simply look into each other's eyes without saying a word. Resist the temptation to make funny faces or sounds. Notice what comes up for you in doing this. Are you tempted to make each other laugh? Do you feel like you need to smile even though that's not how you feel? Do you feel afraid? Is there a longing or sadness that comes up? Are you filled with love and appreciation? Whatever is there, just make a mental note of it. When the timer goes off, you can share with each other what came up for you in the exercise. The next exercise is an excellent format to do that in.

 Fact

> A very important part of attachment for babies is looking into their caregiver's eyes and sensing the emotional bond and the connection there. Because a baby is completely dependent on her caregiver for survival, mutual eye gazing with a caregiver helps build trust that her needs will be met.

Soul Sharing

Soul sharing is a chance to share what is most alive in your soul with a lover or a friend. New lovers may do this naturally, as they are just getting to know each other. But this should never stop, because life is not stagnant. No matter how long you have been with a lover or how well you may think you know each other, life's tides are always changing. It is important to keep checking in to see how the water is.

Soul sharing is about expressing what is in your heart and on your mind. It could be about your hopes, dreams, and visions, or fears, doubts, and concerns for the future. What you share could pertain to current events in your life that are bringing you either joy or frustration. It could be sharing what you are grateful for, or what you really wish wasn't happening in your life.

Soul sharing requires that you first do some self-reflection to get in touch with what is going on for you. To start, sit quietly and focus your attention inward. Shut off the part of your brain that is making lists of things for you to do, judging yourself or others, or wishing you were somewhere else doing something else. You need to get underneath all of that brain activity and tap into the world of your soul, the place where your heart, body, and mind converge.

For this exercise, give yourselves at least twenty to thirty minutes and no more than an hour. Sit directly across from each other, either on the floor or in chairs, whichever is more comfortable. Place a candle between the two of you. Spend a few minutes in self-reflection, during which time you both remain silent, gazing into the candle flame and looking inward. Then, one of you will choose to share by pulling the candle toward you. You will both continue to gaze into the candle's flame while one of you talks about your experience.

 Essential

When sharing, be careful not to use language that may hurt your lover. Share from your heart in a non-blaming way. The listener simply takes it in and does not respond. You are just gathering information about your lover's experience. There is nothing you need to do or say as the listener.

When the first person is done sharing, she will slide the candle toward her partner. Both partners may momentarily look into each other's eyes without saying anything, just acknowledging what has been said. Then it will be the second person's turn. Again, start by taking a little time before speaking to self-reflect and come back into your own experience. Resist any urge to respond to the first person's share. Go inside and find your own truth. Once the second person has shared, push the candle back into the center of the space between you. Then look into each other's eyes again and silently acknowledge the share.

CHAPTER 7

The Art of Sensuality

S ensuality is defined as the gratification of the senses. Sexual pleasure is, of course, one kind of gratification. But really sensual sex can involve a whole lot more. Indulging all of your senses in pleasure is a way to bring more of yourself on board for your arousal and orgasm. Attention to your senses can help you enjoy all the notes your body-instrument can play. The more kinds of sensual pleasure you experience, the richer and more satisfying your lovemaking will be.

Creating a Sensual Environment

Creating a sensual environment is a good way to set the stage for your romantic and sexual encounters. Think of your home, or at least one room in your home, as your love nest. A sensual nest is a place where you can totally relax and enjoy yourself. Putting some extra effort into making your home, or your bedroom, a beautiful, serene, and sensual environment has the potential to greatly increase your enjoyment of the erotic interactions that take place there.

A Clean and Clutter-Free Home

The first step in creating your sensual love sanctuary is to clean your home and clear it of any clutter. A clean and clutter-free home feels fresh. It is a space that allows you to relax because there are no messes or unfinished tasks to distract you. If cleaning your whole home is a daunting task, just focus on your bedroom. Make it a place where you mind is clear enough to really enjoy your body.

Adding Pleasing Colors and Textures

Decorate your love nest. Have fun by adding some sensual colors and textures to the environment. You can do this by painting a wall or two, reupholstering a chair or sofa, getting a new bedspread, or putting up new blinds, drapes, or curtains. Choose colors and textures that attract you and make you feel good. Allow yourself to be bold. Express yourself!

Soft Romantic Lighting

Lighting is essential in creating a romantic mood in your home. Overhead lights, unless they are on dimmers, might not do much for your romantic setting. Spaces and people generally look better in soft lighting. Adding some accent lamps to your home will keep the ambiance more relaxed and laid back. Oil lamps and candles are nice to have for special occasions.

 Alert

In choosing finishing touches, less is more. Don't create more clutter in the process of attempting to beautify your space. Choose only items you love, not just items you think would look good in the space. You should have a positive emotional reaction to any item you bring into your love nest.

Beautiful Finishing Touches

Finally, adding artwork and flowers that you find particularly beautiful and inspiring in some way will add significantly to the enjoyment of your space. These accents also have the potential to bring more color and texture into your home. In choosing finishing touches, consider the whole space and the mood you want to create. Choose items that will enhance that mood and make the space even more pleasing to you.

Sensual Massage

Sensual massage is a perfect way to indulge in the sense of touch. It is also a very effective way to build arousal, whether you are giving or receiving the massage. The use of oil or lotion lightly stroked across your lover's sensuous bare skin is almost guaranteed to get her juices flowing. Sensual massage will help your lover relax and feel good in her body. It will also help her feel loved and cared for. You don't need to be a professional to make your lover feel good. In fact, you have the benefit of being her lover, which means you are in the position to make her feel really good.

What You'll Need

To give a full body massage to your lover, you will need a flat, comfortable surface—like the floor or a bed—a sheet or towel, some massage oil or lotion, and a pillow or rolled up towel. If you have difficulty being on your knees, you may consider using a massage table. Massage tables allow the person giving the massage to stand comfortably. They also usually have a face cradle, which is often more comfortable for the person receiving the massage.

Preparing for the Massage

Make sure you prepare time before the massage to adequately heat the space. If you have a fireplace or woodstove, light a fire to eat up the space and create a cozy atmosphere. Otherwise set the thermostat to anywhere between 75° and 85°F. Light some candles and put some nice relaxing music on. Heat up the massage oil and lotion by setting the bottles in some hot water. Set up the massage table with sheets or lay a towel or sheet on the bed or floor.

Check in with Your Lover

Before you start the massage, check in with your lover about any sore or tight areas in his body that you can send some love to. Find out how much pressure your lover prefers. Once you have checked in, have your lover start by lying face down on the massage table, bed, or floor. Place a pillow, bolster, or rolled up towel under his ankles. Ask if he prefers that or nothing.

 Alert

> Oil is likely to stain the sheet or towel, so make sure you choose something appropriate for this use. Consider keeping some old sheets or towels and designating them for massage. This can help keep you from ruining your other sheets and towels.

Start with Light Caressing

To begin, lightly caress your lover's entire body. Alternate between using your whole hand and just your fingertips. Start with the back and the arms. Then move down to include both legs and feet. If you tend to have sweaty palms, or if there is moisture on your lover's body, light caressing can be challenging, as the hands will tend to get stuck on the skin rather than glide. To remedy this, you can simply throw a soft sheet over your lover's body, and caress him over the sheet.

Begin the Oil or Lotion Massage

To begin using lubrication, place about a tablespoon of warm oil or lotion in your hand. Then rub your hands together to allow the oil to coat the entire surface of both palms. Kneeling or standing at her head, bring both hands gently down onto either side of her spine, and use soft, broad, flowing strokes to move from the top of her back to the small of her back. Then glide your hands across the small of her back, over her hips. For your return stroke, pull your palms up the sides of her body, gliding underneath her armpits and across her shoulder blades to the base of her neck. Additionally, you can stroke down along the top of her shoulders and then back up to the neck. Repeat these strokes many times, improvising on the pattern if you wish.

 Fact

> The use of essential oils in products tends to be the least overbearing and most pleasing to the olfactory system. If you use scented candles, oil, or lotion, make sure you and your lover agree on the scent. Many people have slightly allergic reactions to certain chemicals used in scented products; if you or your lover is sensitive to these, test the product on a small area before progressing to a full body massage.

You can gradually begin to extend your stroke to cover the buttocks and up the sides of the hips. The return stroke can extend over the shoulders and down the arms. Keep the flow going, changing directions seamlessly, eventually covering every inch of your lover's body. Add oil or lotion as needed to keep your hands gliding nicely over her skin. Make sure your hands remain in full contact with your partner's skin during these strokes, molding them to her body in a relaxed manner. Keep the pace slow and occasionally check in with her about the both the pace and the pressure.

When you are ready, move down to the legs. First apply the oil with gentle strokes. Then, starting at the ankle, glide over the calf, across the back of the knee, up the hamstrings, and over the buttocks. In the same stroke, continue all the way up the side of the back, over the shoulder and down the arm on the same side. This long stroke connects the whole body and helps keep the energy flowing. You can do this stroke many times and occasionally work smaller sections by gliding back and forth over the skin in rhythmic, wave-like patterns. Repeat this stroke on the other side. Remember to keep your hands relaxed, the pace slow and sensual, and the pressure to your lover's liking.

The Front of the Body

Once you have worked the left and right sides of the back of your lover's body, gently ask your lover to turn over onto her back in order to massage the front of her body. You can begin by lightly caressing all over the front of her body, as you did on her backside. When you are ready to move on, put another tablespoon of oil onto your hands and begin at the ankle of one leg, gliding over the shin and knee and across the top of the thigh. When you get to the top of the leg crease, swoop your hands to either side of the thigh, and come back down the sides of the leg, all the way to the ankle. Repeat this stroke, making sure to touch all parts of the leg, keeping the pressure light and the strokes flowing and sensual. Repeat these strokes on the other leg.

 Essential

During the sensual massage, allow your fingers to come close your lover's genitals and even linger ever so briefly in the vicinity, but don't actually touch them. The inner thighs and groin creases are exquisitely sensitive, and you can build up a lot of sexual tension just by stroking these parts. This will help build a sense of anticipation.

Once you have massaged both legs, stand or kneel by the top of your lover's head. Rub some oil into your hands. When massaging a female lover, ask what kind of touch, if any, she would like on her breasts during the massage. Then, starting at the top of her chest, gently apply the oil to her torso. Stroke down across the chest, breasts, and abdomen, out to either side. Let your return stroke come up the sides, underneath the armpits, up over the chest, and out the tops of the shoulders. Repeat this stroke many times, making it as slow and delicious as you possibly can. Gradually extend this stroke by gliding from the shoulders all the way down the arms and back up to the neck. Cover as much of her torso as you can.

Stay Present

Throughout the massage, remember to keep checking in with your lover about the pressure and the pace. Keep your touch relatively light, smooth, and flowing. Allow yourself to get turned on while giving the massage. Bring your sexual energy into it, but don't let it override your primary focus of providing a slow sensual experience for your lover. Help her relax and deepen into the pleasure without any feeling of pressure to take care of your needs. Even if she starts to get really turned on, patiently maintain the slow and sensual quality of the massage. She may start to writhe in erotic pleasure underneath your hands or she may deepen her relaxation. Either way, maintain a sensual tone with your touch.

Skin Delicious

Your skin is an erogenous zone. Awakening the skin all over your body can bring more arousal to the rest of your body, but it can also be an ecstatic experience in and of itself. There are many ways to delight in the communion and sensuousness of touching skin. Sensual massage is just one. This section outlines some other possibilities.

Sensual Shower

Showering together can be a very sensuous experience. The feel of warm or hot water combined with slippery soap and your lover's skin can create a very playful and erotic encounter for the two of you. Take turns rubbing each other up and down with a nicely scented soap or shower gel. Make sure you give each other a very thorough cleaning, getting into all the cracks and crevices: behind the ears, under the arms, between the butt cheeks, and even between the toes! Lather each other up simultaneously or one at a time, using hands and other body parts to spread suds on your partner's body. Enjoy the slipping and sliding of your skin against your lover's.

Rub-a-Dub-Dub in the Tub

Taking a bath together can be a very romantic and sensual experience, and it can greatly increase your feelings of intimacy with your lover. Before you get in, add some essential oils to the water for aromatherapy or add bubble bath for fun. Light some candles and put some relaxing music on to create your preferred ambiance. This is a great time to connect and nurture each other. Spend some time facing each other and giving each other foot rubs.

If one of you wants to feel the other's support, then spend some time, facing the same direction, with one of you sitting between the other's legs and resting against your lover's chest. This is a great position for the person behind to wash and caress the upper torso of the person in front. Don't forget to wash each other's backs, necks, and faces. Also, let yourselves be playful, like kids in a bathtub. You might even want to have a rubber ducky or other floating bath toys in there with you.

Mutual Oil Massage and Dance

This sensual play involves covering your body and your lover's body in copious amounts of oil, and then sliding and gliding your bodies across each other in slow and sensual ways that feel good to you. It feels like simultaneously giving and receiving a full body massage. You can use any vegetable oil, but olive oil and coconut oil, slightly warmed, are particularly nice and actually good for the skin. You can also use a massage oil that is lightly scented with essential oils to add a delightful treat for your olfactory system.

 Alert

Be careful and stay safe! Oily skin can get very slippery. Make sure you don't slip and fall onto a hard surface. Choose a soft surface like the grass, a carpeted area, or your bed to play on. This will also be more comfortable when you lie down and begin rolling on top of each other.

To prevent getting oil all over the place, lay down a large sheet of plastic and cover it with an old sheet. Doing this outside in your backyard works well if you have privacy. You can also cover your bed with a vinyl waterproof sheet. Make sure you have a plan for how you will wash off afterward.

Have fun exploring with each other. See how many ways you can slide across your lover's body. Surrender to the sensations, letting every part of your body get some attention. Include even your face and scalp. Let your hair get oily. This is a chance to dive into the sensual pleasure of your flesh. You use your whole body to do this, front and back. Slip and slide your way to bliss with your lover!

The Sensual Art of Kissing

Kissing is truly a sensual art. It is a very popular way of building the heat between lovers. The lips and mouth are highly erogenous for many people. Some women have even claimed to orgasm from kissing alone. Some lovers find they enjoy the act of kissing so much that they could just do this for hours, usually combined with caressing and fondling.

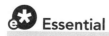 **Essential**

Kissing is a way to begin to explore the merging of your sexual energies. It is how you can begin to listen to each other energetically and create a dance that is all your own. When starting a new sexual connection with someone, spend a fair amount of time just exploring through kissing.

Preparing for Kissing

Kissing is a very personal and intimate act. It can make you feel vulnerable, so it is something for which you want to feel prepared. There are several things you can do to prepare for kissing that will make your kissing encounter more enjoyable. The first is to keep your lips soft and supple. The second is to make sure your breath is not offensive. And the third is to know when the time and circumstances are right.

Caring For Your Lips

Keeping your lips soft and supple will ensure that they feel good to you and your lover. Chapped, dry lips are painful and are not likely to be pleasant for your partner to kiss. To keep your lips soft and supple, drink lots of water. Keeping your body hydrated will help significantly with the quality of your skin in general, including your lips. Also, avoid licking and biting your lips. To keep your lips from becoming chapped and dry, make sure to use an SPF lip protector when out in the sun for long periods of time, and use lip balm to protect your lips when you will be exposed to wind. For extra treatment, you can apply lip balm at night before you go to bed or try exfoliating your lips with a salt or sugar scrub, a loofa sponge or exfoliating glove, or even your toothbrush.

Attend to Your Breath

Being worried about your breath can hinder your enjoyment and experience of kissing your lover. While your lover would hopefully feel comfortable enough telling you your breath was off, you can't necessarily count on that. It is also considerate and practical to take matters into your own hands when it comes to your own breath. Anything you can do to assure that your breath is not offensive will help keep both you and your lover worry-free and happy. Poor digestion, illness, tooth or gum decay, certain foods and beverages, and smoking can all contribute to bad breath. Some of these are obviously more easily remedied than others. You owe it to yourself and your partner to do all that you can to make sure your breath is not going to get in the way of your enjoyment of kissing one another.

Prevention strategies and remedies for bad breath depend upon what is causing the problem. Good practices include the following: Pay attention to the food you eat and your subsequent digestion, consulting a nutritionist if needed. Floss and brush your teeth regularly to keep your mouth free of decay and infection. And finally, scrape your tongue with a tongue scraper. This can be very effective, as it will remove bacteria from the tongue, which is often responsible for bad breath. The use of mouthwash can help too, but not everybody likes the smell of mouthwash.

 Fact

You can self-test your own breath by licking the back of your hand, waiting a few seconds, and then smelling your hand. This will enable you to know exactly what your breath smells like. If it smells fine to you, chances are your lover won't mind either.

If you drink coffee, beer, or other alcohol; smoke; or eat a lot of garlic, you should check it out with your lover to see how his olfactory system responds to these smells, as they do tend to linger on the breath and some people find them unpleasant. You may find that if both you and your lover are drinking beer or eating garlic together, you are not as likely to get offended by those smells. Eating a sprig of parsley after a garlicky meal is said to freshen the breath.

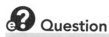 **Question**

What can I do if my lover does not like the smell of something on my breath that I partake in regularly?
Your options are to quit the food or substance altogether or to limit it to times you won't be connecting sexually. You can also try to somehow mask the smell, but be warned that this is often not successful.

Is the Time Right?

You need to be able to read the cues from your lover or lover-to-be to know when the time is right for kissing. For some, kissing is a very private thing and only to be done when the two of you are alone. For others, kissing in public is fun and sexy. Comfort levels can vary depending on the type of kiss and the specific people who may be observing. If you find that you are not sure whether kissing someone is okay in a particular context, it doesn't hurt to ask.

In general, people tend to feel most ready to kiss when they are alone on an intimate date. Establishing a connection by talking and cultivating an emotional closeness can set the stage. You are more likely to be ready to kiss when your bodies are already touching. This could be a casual touch, not necessarily a passionate embrace. You are clearly ready to kiss when you both feel the heat between the two of you.

Becoming a Better Kisser

There is certainly no right or wrong way to kiss. But there are many variations to kissing. While you probably have found a way to kiss that works for you and your lover, you may be open to try some new techniques. Expanding your repertoire gives you more options to draw upon and can help make you a more exciting and versatile lover.

Think about kissing in several different stages. First, there is the approach. Then there is the meeting and discovering of your lips and mouths. Following this is the passionate build-up. And finally, there is the ending of the kiss.

The Approach

When you approach your lover to begin kissing, it is good to be relaxed. Move slowly. You don't want to accidentally bump heads or clash teeth. It can be helpful to just bring your faces close to each other initially and listen and feel each other's breath. Take time to smell and breathe in your lover's hair, skin, and breath. Notice how you are feeling, being this close. Allow your cheeks to brush up against each other if that feels good to you. Allow your lips to softly graze against each other's. Gently explore each other's faces with your lips and nose. Wander off to the sides, exploring each other's ears and necks.

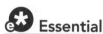 **Essential**

Listen with your whole being. Allow the anticipation and curiosity to build. Don't be in a hurry. Enjoy the approach as if it were very much a part of the kiss. Allow yourself to be moved by the tenderness and vulnerability of connecting on such an intimate level.

Tender Kissing and Nibbling

Tender kissing helps create a feeling of safety. Gentle biting or nibbling is a way to increase excitement while maintaining a feeling of tenderness. Tender kissing and nibbling can either stand on their own or be a prelude to passionate kissing. You can start by planting tender kisses and nibbles on different parts of your lover's face, ears, neck, and shoulders. When your lips first meet, they should be relaxed. You are looking to merge your lips delicately together. Allow your lips to really enjoy the feeling of your lover's lips. Move your lips in a way that feels good, not in a way that you think is supposed to look good. The feeling of sensitivity behind the kissing is what makes it tender. Appreciate the vulnerability of being so close.

Passionate Kissing

Passionate kissing occurs when the heat is really high or when one of you wants to turn it up. People generally equate passionate kissing with French kissing (open mouthed). But passion actually has more to do with the energy behind the kiss, rather than whether your tongue is involved. Stay attentive to your lover even as the passion builds. Be careful not to get swept away by your own arousal, and stop paying attention to your lover's energy. She may be in a very different place, and you may lose her in the kiss.

When you do bring your tongue in on the action, notice your lover's response. Take turns offering your tongue into your lover's mouth. Don't let it turn into a wrestling match between your tongues. Extending your tongue may mean, "I want to be inside of you" or "I want to be closer to you." Let the action stem from your feelings, rather than from a mechanical idea of what kissing is supposed to be.

> **EXERCISE:** Practice your kissing on a succulent fruit, such as a mango. Make sure you choose a fruit you enjoy. Peel away the skin to expose the juicy part of the fruit, and let your lips luxuriate in the sensuous texture and juiciness. Then try kissing your lover in the same way.

Sealing the Kiss

Knowing when to stop kissing can be as challenging as knowing when to start. You may want to stop before you sense your lover is ready. It is best to find a way to transition gradually so that your lover can adjust her energy to the shift. You don't want your lover feeling suddenly abandoned. A good way to transition out of passionate kissing is to go back to tender kissing for a while. Or when you decide to stop kissing, you could express verbally how much you love kissing her or look her in the eyes and smile.

CHAPTER 8

Erotic Play:
Building Up the Heat

Your orgasms will be influenced by how much arousal, sexual heat, or tension you have built up in your body. If you want to increase the potency and quality of your orgasms, you will need to build more sexual tension. There are many ways to play with sexual energy to increase desire and arousal. For some, getting really turned on is the best part. If you haven't put much effort into building arousal in your erotic connections, you may find you have been missing out on a lot of pleasure and fun!

The Art of Seduction

Getting someone interested in having sex with you is an exciting endeavor. Depending on the circumstances, it can be either very easy or completely impossible. Still, you can have fun trying. There are many ways to entice and seduce someone into a sexual encounter with you. Most include somehow conveying that you want to make your potential lover feel really good, whatever it takes. If you can do that with your words, actions, and behaviors, then you are off to a good start. Confidence, born from experience in pleasuring others, will also help, as will being comfortable with your own sexuality. But even if you don't have much experience, fear not, because a willingness to learn can be very seductive.

The Art of Flirting

Flirting is behaving in a sexually enticing way. It can be expressing that you are a vibrant sexual being or that you are sexually interested in someone. It's a fun way to start to get the juices flowing within you, or between you and another person. Flirting behavior includes how you dress, how you make eye contact, how you talk, and what your body language says. You may flirt without even being aware that you are doing it. Sometimes sexual interest lies just under the surface of your conscious recognition.

 Fact

In the Victorian era, women used fans as playful props to send their flirtatious messages. A fan placed near the heart was a signal that the admirer had won the lady's love. A fan pressed to her lips meant her admirer could kiss her. To show she was in love, a lady would hide her eyes behind an open fan.

Dressing Flirtatiously

Flirtatious dressing prompts people to take notice, be attracted, or become curious about you. The way you dress may call attention to certain features on your body or certain attributes of your personality, perhaps your flair for style, color, comfort, or fun. You may be subtle or outrageous. You don't have to dress in a way that says, "Take me to bed this instant!" unless, of course, that's what you want.

To get people to notice certain features on your body, you may wear a piece of jewelry or an article of clothing that accentuates that part. To get them to notice a particular personality trait, you may choose to dress stylishly, expressing your fashion sense, or really colorfully, expressing your love of color. You may choose soft fabrics that beg to be touched, or you may dress in a quirky way to display your uniqueness or your sense of fun. The best way to dress flirtatiously is to express yourself freely.

Eye Contact

Making eye contact with someone is often the first way you express sexual interest. Letting someone catch you looking at him with interest can be very seductive. Maintaining eye contact is uncomfortable for some people, but it is a skill that can be developed. Calm and clear eye contact can express confidence, interest, and availability.

Paradoxically, shyness too can be seductive. In fact, sometimes coyly looking away is very alluring. It may express that you are extremely attracted and just need some help feeling safe enough to show it. Whether you project confidence or coyness, smiling will help you be more seductive. It is hard to resist a face that lights up in a big smile.

Flirtatious Talk

Usually, flirting involves some type of playful or suggestive conversation. Everybody develops her own style, but in general, flirtatious conversation is light, fun, upbeat, and sexy. With flirtatious talk, you may try to convey how desirable you are in clever ways. You may hint that you are a very gifted lover and know your way around a man. Or you may play hard to get. Conversely, you may focus your attention on the person you are flirting with, offering him obvious compliments or flattery. You might make up playful nicknames, engage in good-humored banter, or make a lot of jokes or sexual innuendoes.

 Essential

The trick to flirtatious talk is making sure that whomever you are flirting with is on board with you, not getting offended, and has room to respond. If you are the only one flirting, you might be making a fool of yourself or just being a nuisance. Be sensitive to your audience, but by all means, have fun!

Body Language

Whether you are aware of it or not, your body language could give off signals that you are sexually interested in someone. If you become aware of what kind of body language expresses sexual interest, you can use it to help you flirt and build up the heat within yourself and/or between you and another person. Awareness of your body language can also keep you from sending the wrong message to someone you are not interested in.

You can also use your body language to draw attention to parts of your body that you think are sexy. You can play with your hair, brushing it back with your fingers or tucking it behind your ear. You can cross and uncross your legs slowly, or do things to call attention to your mouth or neck, like bite or lick your lips or rub or touch your neck. You can stretch your arms up in the air and draw attention to your underarms. You can nonchalantly open an article of clothing and expose some bare skin. Whether or not you deliberately use body language to flirt, it can be interesting to try to notice if you also use it unconsciously at times.

 Alert

Flirting isn't always intended to be sexual. But it can sometimes be challenging to differentiate between friendliness and sexual interest. You may be someone or know someone who flirts for the sake of flirting, without any real interest in taking an interaction further. Some people flirt just to spice up a conversation, feel attractive, or get some attention.

Building Sexual Tension

Sexual tension is the energy that builds inside of you, making you yearn for sexual release or orgasm. Sometimes the build-up of this energy is very strong and occurs automatically, without any conscious effort. But this is not the case for everyone. You may need to put some effort into building sexual tension in order to enjoy high levels of arousal, sexual release, and orgasm.

Sexual tension is usually a product of the interaction between people. It is especially high when both people are strongly attracted to each other. Strong sexual tension seems to be naturally built into certain relationships. In others, it needs to be consciously cultivated. Sexual tension is created when there are both feelings of safety and fear. A feeling of safety makes it so that you can relax into a sexual encounter. A little bit of fear is what makes a sexual encounter exciting. New sexual relationships usually have fear built into them because there is always fear in the unknown. Long-term relationships may have plenty of familiarity and safety, but sometimes there is not enough fear to keep the sexual tension alive without conscious effort.

 Fact

The more sexual tension builds up, the greater and more exciting the sexual release. Learn how to work with sexual tension by introducing a little bit of fear into the mix when that is lacking. Cultivate feelings of safety if that is what is necessary. This can help you keep the sexual music you make together dynamic and exciting.

In the art of seduction, you learn to take your time to let the energy build between you and your lover. Many lovers have a habit of going directly for sexual release or gratification. They use only whatever sexual energy exists in them when they first get together, rather than allowing the erotic energy or tension between them to build over time. Regardless of how long you have been with a lover, it is important to keep the art of seduction alive if you want to ensure that the fires keep burning.

Dressing Up (or Down) to Seduce

Dressing up can be a fun and creative way to turn up the heat between you and your lover. When you wear something that is different from your ordinary attire, you introduce a new and exciting element. Playing with your wardrobe is something you can do for its own erotic appeal, or to supplement other kinds of erotic play, such as erotic dancing and role-playing.

Your Birthday Suit

When was the last time you pranced around the house naked? Nudity is very sexy. Wearing nothing but your birthday suit can be a real turn on for both of you. Flesh is beautiful, and having it all out in the open can feel very inviting. If you are someone who loves the feeling of your own bare flesh up against someone else's bare flesh, this can be absolutely intoxicating. There is no fabric that can quite compare to the sensuous look and feel of the bare skin of your lover.

Nudity also offers an element of raw vulnerability. Who you are when you are naked is who you are in your most raw form. You may prefer to cover yourself up, because being naked feels scary. But allowing yourself to be seen in your raw form can increase a sense of intimacy. It can be very liberating. And it can add to the sexual tension between you and your lover. Don't underestimate the power of your naked self.

Costumes

Costumes don't have to be just for Halloween. Dressing up in costumes is a great way to add some fun and extra creativity to your sex life. Wearing a costume facilitates the exploration of different parts of yourself and can even help you feel like another person altogether. Costumes can help you start fun role-plays. You can draw on your fantasy life for ideas of costumes that might turn you and your lover on.

Here are some classic ideas for costumes to consider:

- Angel or Devil
- Athlete/Cheerleader
- Butler/Maid
- Courtly lovers
- Cowgirl/Cowboy
- Goddess/God
- Kitty Cat/Wild Cat
- Law Enforcement/Military
- Maintenance/Fixer-upper guy
- Nurse/Doctor
- Pirate/Swashbuckler
- Professor/Teacher
- Prostitute/Pimp
- Sailor
- Schoolgirl/Schoolboy

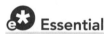 **Essential**

When shopping with a lover for sexy underwear or lingerie, be sure that whatever you choose makes you feel sexy and doesn't just please her. If she gets really turned on by something you try on for her, you could let that influence how sexy you feel. Make sure your decisions make both of you happy.

Sexy Underwear and Lingerie

Sexy underwear and lingerie are staples in sexy attire. They come in soft and silky fabrics. They can accentuate particular aspects of your form. They may reveal a lot of flesh, and/or teasingly conceal certain body parts. When purchasing these items, make sure that you try them on first. This allows you to gauge how well they fit and whether they feel good on you. You can surprise your lover by secretly wearing lingerie underneath your clothing and then revealing it at some point, perhaps during a strip tease. Or you can both go shopping, trying things on and choosing your selections together.

Erotic Talk

Using words to get turned on or to turn your lover on is often very fun. Since the brain is ultimately responsible for sexual arousal and orgasm, the use of language to stimulate the brain can be a surprisingly direct route to arousal. There are many ways that you can turn your lover on with words.

Talking Dirty

Graphic descriptions of how turned on you are and all the things you want to do with your lover can lend your lovemaking an edge of assertiveness, aggressiveness, raunchiness, or bawdiness. This boldness is part of what makes talking dirty so seductive. This is also what can make it embarrassing or scary.

It can be helpful to ask your partner how she feels about graphic language. It can be a relief to know if you have a green light in this department. And it is important to know if there are any limits for either of you. If dirty talk works for both you and your lover, then get creative and have fun with it!

Sexy E-mails, Text Messages, Erotic Letters, and Love Poems

Sending your lover a sexy e-mail, text message, letter, or poem is a great way to express your desire and turn up the heat between the two of you. It can be a wonderful prelude to a date later on that evening or it can be something you do between dates to keep the juices flowing. You may feel bolder and more creative when it comes to expressing your erotic feelings in writing. This is also a great way to set the stage for any fantasies or role-plays that you may want to act out later.

Phone Sex

Hearing your lover's voice on the phone can be the ultimate in foreplay. He is so close and yet so far. Because you can't actually touch, phone sex offers a chance to slow the action down. You can really learn to appreciate the power of language when a verbal connection is all you have to work with. If you have to be apart from your lover, phone sex can take the place of being able to connect physically with one another.

When having phone sex with your lover, try closing your eyes. Let yourself feel the desire to be with him in person, or imagine that you are together. Say all the things you want to do and all the ways he turns you on. Feel the sexual tension build. Use that feeling of desire and longing to fuel what you say and how you say it. Sighing and moaning, whispering your desires, and talking dirty are all likely to build the energy between the two of you. Feel free to self-pleasure while you converse.

Erotic Touch

Erotic touch is any kind of touch that results in sexual arousal. Both men and women respond to erotic touch, but what turns each person on varies. You will have to explore different kinds of touch to see what works for your lover. You can always ask her how she likes to be touched or suggest ways that you would like to touch her and see how she responds. Learning how to skillfully touch your lover in a way that makes her sexually aroused or increases her arousal is a key to being a good lover.

Caressing

Caressing expresses tenderness and creates a sense of intimacy and safety. Light, gentle stokes of your hand on your partner's body can encourage relaxation and surrender. It can also potentially lead to arousal, given the right circumstances.

There are numerous ways to caress and many parts of the body that like to be caressed. You can use just your fingertips, your whole hand, or the back of your hand. It is nice to combine all of these for variety. Generally, caressing feels best when done with a relaxed hand at a slow pace. Start by caressing the face and neck, the upper chest, shoulders and arms, the back, particularly the small of the back, and possibly the belly. Then, extend your caresses to your partner's erogenous zones and start building the heat.

 Alert

If you have very rough hands, it may not feel good to your lover to use your fingertips or the palm of your hand for caressing. You can try the back of your hand or use a feather, a feather duster, or a fuzzy mitten. The soft touch of these can feel divine.

Pinching and Grabbing

Pinching and grabbing involve using your fingers or your whole hand to grab onto and squeeze a fleshy part of your partner's body. It expresses passion and desire and can be very effective at helping to build sexual tension. Not everyone likes pinching and grabbing, and it is only appropriate at certain times. It is usually best when there is already a fair amount of arousal built up, or if you are both in a playful mood.

The buttocks, nipples, clitoris, and labia (gently) are particularly responsive to pinching. The erect penis, the arms, the hips, the buttocks, and the breasts are generally responsive to grabbing. As with everything you do with your lover, and especially with rougher erotic behaviors, it is a good idea to check in about the desired quality and quantity.

Teasing

Teasing touch is another way to create a feeling of yearning and desire. Good teasing is all about finding desire's edge and dancing back and forth across it. There's an art to building the fire in someone, letting it cool a little, and building it again and again and again. It slowly raises the passion to a new plateau.

Teasing may involve touching a little bit and then withdrawing completely or varying the kind of touch or the place you touch. For some people teasing the genitals is a very effective way to build up arousal. This can be done by touching all around the genitals but not on them directly. Another way is to lightly stimulate the genitals at irregular intervals. It can be fun to see how much teasing you can take and how much arousal you can build up with teasing alone.

Spanking

Spanking can be either light patting or hard smacking on the buttocks. There seems to be a bit of a spanking craze right now. More and more people are getting into this naughty delight. If you have never tried it but think it might work for you, there is no time like the present. Spanking can be done on a clothed or a bare bottom. You can be standing, bending over, or lying down. The skin on the behind is very sensitive and because of the proximity to the genitals, it is particularly erotic. Tension can start to build in the buttocks and the whole pelvic region with the anticipation of each slap. It can be especially effective at building arousal when combined with a fantasy or role-play.

Dancing

Dancing with a lover is a great way to build up the heat. Dancing puts you into your body and gets your energy moving. Energetic dancing can release endorphins, your body's "feel good" hormones. When you dance, let yourself be inspired and moved by the music in ways that feel really good to you. If you are feeling good in your body, you probably look good to your lover.

There are many ways to bring dancing into your erotic life. In addition to going out and dancing at concerts, clubs, or other venues, you can clear a space in your living room or bedroom for some private dancing action. You can use dirty dancing, erotic dancing, lap dancing, and strip teasing to get the juices flowing.

Dirty Dancing

Dirty dancing is a way to let the sexual energy between you and another person influence how you move together on the floor. Dirty dancing tends to be very focused on the pelvis. It may include a lot of bumping and grinding. Your whole body is usually touching and moving with your partner, enjoying the heat between you. Feel each other's muscles and flesh and try to merge your movements. If you are a woman, you can straddle your lover's leg and feel your clitoris rubbing against it. If you are a man, don't be afraid to have an erection and to let your lover know that you have one. Feeling your lover's genitals rubbing against you while dancing can be a huge turn-on!

Erotic Dancing

Erotic dancing is dance performance that involves posturing and moving your body in seductive ways. You can either do this by yourself to help increase your own arousal, or you can dance with your lover. Erotic dancing can be very arousing to both the performer and the audience. Whether you are a man or a woman, you should consider adding this delightful treat to your erotic repertoire.

The most important elements of erotic dancing are expressing your sexiness and having fun. Erotic dancing is about strutting your stuff. Displaying sexual confidence increases your sexual desirability. Showing your partner that you feel good about what you've got to offer is more important than having the right shape or the right moves. You need to be able to turn off your critical mind and have fun.

Erotic Dancing Techniques

Regardless of whether you are a man or a woman, there are some universal techniques that can help make your erotic dancing particularly hot. First of all, dress in a sexy and revealing way. This will get your lover's attention immediately. When it comes to posturing, think suggestive. You want to draw attention to the sexualized parts of your body, like your butt, your chest or breasts, and your pelvis. Slowing your movement down can help build the tension. Crawling on the floor toward your lover like a cat or a wild animal on the prowl can be very sexy. Try snarling and growling like an animal to release more primal passions. Smiling seductively or coyly can also be a real turn on. You can occasionally speed up the movement for added excitement. Try suddenly thrusting your pelvis up and down several times. This may take your lover by surprise and increase the sexual tension.

 Alert

If you are not having fun doing your erotic dance, then something is definitely not right. This should be enjoyable and you should do it because you want to, not just because you think it will please your lover. It can be a little scary if it's new for you, but you can still have fun with it. If it is not your thing, that's okay too.

Masculine Suggestions

If you want to display your masculine strength and power, move in a way that stretches and flexes your muscles a lot. Gyrate and thrust your hips and pelvis. Displaying your ability to move that part of your body will surely get your lover to take notice.

Feminine Suggestions

If you want to display your feminine prowess, try arching your lower back so that your butt sticks out some. Keep your chest and breasts jutting out and your shoulders down and back. And keep at least one leg completely straight when standing. Think of a filly trotting. This posturing puts it all out there on display, in a prideful way. Also, keep your toes pointed. This extension creates tension in the legs that your lover will likely find enticing.

Lap Dancing

Lap dancing is erotic dance with the added bonus of physically connecting with your audience. Generally, the one who is receiving the lap dance is not allowed to touch the dancer. This restriction helps build the sexual tension. Sometimes, the dancer also refrains from actual touch, but comes palpably close. You can set up your own guidelines for a lap dance with your lover. Although it is usually thought of as something women do, there is no reason why men can't offer lap dances too. As with erotic dancing, it helps to dress in a suggestive way, exposing a significant amount of flesh. The music you play should be erotic and help you get in the mood.

To begin, set up a chair with no arms for your lover to sit in. Place the chair where there is space to move all around it. Begin by dancing erotically in front of your lover. Allow the tension to build before coming into close physical contact with him. When you feel ready to engage physically with your lover, begin by brushing up lightly against him with different parts of your scantily clad body. Tease your lover with your body. Make your lover want to grab you. When you are ready, try straddling his lap, facing him. Perch your hands on the back of the chair. Then gyrate your hips, bumping and grinding away to the music. You can gently remind him not to touch. Make the dance feel good to you. This is an excellent way for you to get yourself worked up too. You are in control of how to move your pelvis and where to touch him in ways that feel good to you. For variety, you can also straddle your lover facing away from him.

Strip Teasing

A strip tease combines erotic dancing with the art of removing your clothing. Prepare for a strip tease by dressing in carefully planned layers. Include accessories, like a hat, gloves, belt, or scarf, so that you have more to remove, thereby prolonging the experience. The layer closest to your skin might be your favorite sexy underwear or lingerie. The next layer could be a form-fitting outfit or a costume.

Start the performance by getting into a groove with music that you find particularly juicy and erotic. When you sense you have your lover's full attention, you can begin, ever so slowly and gradually, to remove articles of clothing and accessories. The idea is to expose just a little bit of flesh at a time, so take your time with it. As you remove an article, find some sexy way to play with it before throwing it across the room or toward your lover, or letting it drop to the floor.

 Essential

Your dancing and seductive moves are a part of what makes the strip-tease experience sexually arousing. If you are really into your strip-tease and your performance turns you on, then your lover is more likely to get turned on watching you.

Sharing Fantasies and Role-Play

Fantasy enactment and role-playing are excellent ways to increase the heat between you and your lover. Start by each describing one or more of your fantasies. Remember to give yourself and your partner lots of permission to fantasize about things you would never want to do in reality. You may feel vulnerable sharing a fantasy that embarrasses you. But sharing your fantasies is an important way to keep your sex life vibrant and alive. Hearing your partner's fantasies might also feed your own imagination.

Once you have identified some fantasies, you can decide together which ones you might want to act out in a role-play. Role-playing can allow you to experience the excitement of your fantasy in more vivid detail. It is still not real, because you are acting, but it can start to feel very real. Adding costumes to your fantasy and role-play will add an even greater sense of the fantasy coming to life.

Role-playing is a great way to add some sexual tension. Fear often plays an important role in fantasies. Fantasies often, but not always, involve some kind of status or power imbalance. This discrepancy in status or power creates tension. Sometimes fantasies are strictly taboo and that's what makes them exciting. Again, the fear factor adds to the excitement. Different people are drawn to different types of fantasies and role-plays. Here are some common themes to explore, if they sound interesting to you.

Wild Animal and Prey

This fantasy/role-play is for anyone who likes the thrill of the chase. In this role-play, one of you is the hunter and one of you is the prey. The hunter animal gets to be a wild aggressive animal that is hungrily chasing and outwitting its prey. The prey gets to be the fearful helpless object of the hunter's desires. This role-play will likely get you out of the bed and the bedroom and into other parts of the house as the hunter animal tracks down its vulnerable prey.

Teacher and Student

This fantasy/role-play is for anyone who has ever had a crush on or fantasized about being sexual with her teacher. In this fantasy/role-play, one of you is the teacher and one of you is the student. The teacher has more status and is older and wiser. The student is younger and more naive and vulnerable and has something to learn. In this fantasy, the teacher uses her status to seduce the student into a sexual encounter with her.

Sex Worker and John (or Jane)

This fantasy is for anyone who has ever fantasized about paying for sex or being paid for sex. In this fantasy/role-play, one of you is paid to have sex with the other one. You might set it up so that you meet somewhere in public and pay real money before going home. If you want to make it feel even more real, get a hotel room somewhere.

Any of the ideas and activities in this chapter can be used to increase sexual tension and build arousal. The more time you spend with this, the more prepared you will be to experience satisfying orgasms. But the things you do to turn up the heat are really enjoyable themselves. So linger in these build-up activities and enjoy all they have to offer.

CHAPTER 9

You Deserve a Hand: Manual Paths to Orgasm with a Lover

Using your hands is a very natural, effective, and satisfying way to bring yourself or your lover to orgasm. The hands have amazing dexterity and are capable of providing tremendous pleasure. Whether you are self-pleasuring with your lover or using your hands to stimulate each other, you have the capacity to make some beautiful music this way. The love you make with your hands is indeed capable of holding its own when compared to the other paths to orgasm.

Self-Pleasuring with Your Lover

Self-pleasuring with your lover combines all the benefits of masturbation with the excitement and comfort the presence of your lover can offer. Still, many people are embarrassed by the idea or wonder what the point is. If you feel uncomfortable at the notion of self-pleasuring with a lover, consider the following reasons why opening to this idea might be a rewarding way to stretch your mind and improve your sex life.

Taboos and Myths Getting in the Way

It is no wonder that you might feel embarrassed about touching yourself when you are with a lover. Our culture's taboo on masturbation makes touching your own genitals for pleasure shameful at any time, not just when you are alone. But you need not abide by this taboo. You have a right to touch your own body whenever you have the privacy and the desire. You may also suffer from the myth that an orgasm is supposed to be achieved by other some means. Therefore, if you have to use your hands, you are somehow failing. This is as ludicrous as claiming that there is one best flavor of ice cream. There are many ways to have an orgasm. Orgasms that come from your hand or your partner's hand can be just as delicious as any other kind.

Overcoming Shyness or Inhibitions

There is no good reason why touching yourself in front of your lover should be off limits. Unfortunately, many people feel shy about this. Setting an intention to overcome your inhibitions about self-pleasuring while with a lover could be the greatest gift you ever give to your sex life. This is one of those hurdles that has the potential to liberate your sexuality in ways you never imagined possible.

 Fact

Studies have shown that more women are likely to orgasm from manual stimulation alone than from intercourse or oral sex. Combine manual stimulation with intercourse or oral sex, and the chances of a woman having an orgasm with these activities increases significantly. These facts should make it worth overcoming any resistances you may feel.

In order to overcome any shyness, remind yourself that freedom to self-pleasure is something that will contribute to your enjoyment of sex and ultimately your lover's enjoyment too. You may also want to talk with your lover about any scared or vulnerable feelings you have about masturbating in front of him. He may be able to reassure you that he sees nothing wrong with it. It may even turn him on. And finally, you will need to determine the right situations in which you can explore self-pleasuring with your lover.

Assistance from Your Lover

Sometimes it's just nice to have company when you self-pleasure. Your lover can cuddle you or provide stimulation to your other erogenous zones while you take charge of your genitals. If your lover wants to be sexual when you don't, you might still be able to support him while he masturbates. You can kiss his head, stroke his chest, or look into his eyes and tell him how sexy he is and how much you love him.

> **EXERCISE:** Take turns self-pleasuring with each other. When you are the one self-pleasuring, talk with your lover about what you are doing, what you like, and how it feels. When you are supporting, kiss, stroke, and fondle your lover. Spend some time watching closely to see exactly what she is doing with her genitals.

Educating Your Lover

Self-pleasuring in front of your lover is a great way to educate him about how you like to be touched. It is also an excellent way for lovers to learn about each other's sexual response. Even if your lover has had previous lovers and has lots of experience with manual stimulation, your body and preferences are unique, and therefore, she will need to spend time learning about you. As you are self-pleasuring, it can be helpful to describe the finer details of what you are doing that may be difficult to observe. For example, you may want to express the importance of having just the right amount of lubrication. Or, you may want to share that you are touching yourself with the lightest touch possible. Perhaps you like to change what you are doing every few strokes. Don't be shy about sharing with your lover what works for you. This will ultimately help him be a better lover for you, something you will both enjoy.

Self-Pleasuring with Your Lover as Foreplay

Self-pleasuring is a quick and often a sure way of getting your juices flowing. It can jump-start your arousal and help get you in the mood and ready for other sexual activities with a lover. You can kiss and fondle each other's other erogenous zones, while you each stimulate your own genitals just enough to build some arousal in your body. Touching yourself is the most direct way to prepare yourself for intercourse or other sexual behavior that may benefit from higher levels of arousal.

Simultaneous Self-Pleasuring to Achieve Orgasm

Self-pleasuring alongside a lover who is also self-pleasuring has several appealing aspects. First, it is the safest possible way to have sex, since it involves no possibility of bodily fluid exchange. Secondly, if you are pressed for time, masturbation might be the quickest way for both of you to orgasm. And thirdly, it is an interesting way to try something new and different. You can lie next to each other, maybe kissing, or caressing each other with your free hands. Alternatively, you can sit or stand facing each other. This gives you both full visual access to each other's bodies. As you look at each other, let yourselves feel your desire. Combine this with erotic talk or fantasy and you are sure to find a new path to ecstasy that you may choose to visit frequently!

 Essential

It is possible to really connect energetically and make love with your lover while you are each self-pleasuring. Look into each other's eyes, breathe together, and see how much you can feel each other. Let your partner in energetically as you stimulate your own genitals.

Self-Pleasuring to Assist in Orgasm

You may need some assistance in order to orgasm during sex with a lover. This is particularly true with women, whose primary route to orgasm is the clitoris, which does not always get adequately stimulated during particular sexual behaviors. Some men may also need to manually stimulate themselves to maintain their erection or achieve orgasm during different sexual behaviors. Self-pleasuring can be used to speed things up when time is a factor. And it is handy when one person is exhausted before the other is satisfied. Whatever your reason, you should feel no guilt or shame for wanting or needing to touch yourself to enhance your sexual experience.

Manual Stimulation

The general term for using your hand to stimulate your partner's genitals is manual stimulation. The more common slang terms for this are hand job (typically used to refer to giving a man manual pleasure, although can be used for women too) or fingering (pleasuring a woman's vulva and vagina with your fingers). You can take turns giving and receiving manual stimulation or you can give and receive simultaneously. Because the hands and fingers have such fine coordination, some people prefer manual stimulation above all other sexual behaviors.

 Alert

The safety of manual stimulation is not absolute. If your hand has an open cut, then semen or vaginal secretions you touch could come into contact with your blood. Thus, it is possible to get a sexually transmitted disease from giving or receiving manual stimulation, although it is unlikely. Take appropriate precautions. Use latex or vinyl gloves, a condom, or a dental dam if there is any doubt.

Receiving Manual Stimulation

When receiving manual stimulation, it is helpful if you can give your lover preliminary suggestions on how to best touch your genitals. Let him know when you really like what he's doing, and when something he's doing is either hurting or not effective at building your arousal. Often this can be done without words. Let yourself make noise as you are receiving his touch. This can give your lover an immediate feedback loop to work with. When you make a pleasurable sound, it means "do more of that!"

Receiving touch feels best when you relax and surrender as much as you can. This can be a challenge for some people. Tell yourself that you deserve some time to simply enjoy receiving. The more you can let go, the more pleasure you are likely to enjoy, and the more you are likely to experience profound and satisfying orgasms.

Checking in with Your Lover

Offering your hands to pleasure your lover is a real gift. Before you start, ask about any specific likes or dislikes your lover may have. Find out if she has any particular recipe for orgasm through manual stimulation. It's always good to get tips from the expert (your lover) when it comes to her orgasm. If your lover does not have much experience receiving manual stimulation, then you can just try different things while asking her about what works and what doesn't. Continue to check in occasionally as you go along to see if you could change anything you're doing to increase her arousal or facilitate orgasm.

The Approach

In general, your approach should be gentle and you should play close attention to the delicate tissues of the genitals. This will help your lover feel safe to surrender his genitals to your manipulation of them. At the same time, your touch should be confident, allowing your lover to just relax and enjoy, giving him the sense that he is in competent hands. Your initial contact with your lover's bare genitals will set the stage for his being able to surrender to the pleasure you are about to bestow. Your touch should communicate that you really want him to enjoy himself and that you are here to help.

 Fact

Your first touch to your lover's genitals may actually happen over clothes. It could be a gentle brushing or stroking or more of a passionate grabbing or squeezing. This can spark your lover's arousal, but it is not likely to be the thing that brings him to orgasm. For that you will need to do a little more work!

Manual Stimulation Tips for Him and Her

There is no right way to stimulate your lover's genitals with your hands. Each person will have her own particular desires and preferences for manual stimulation. But there are some general tips and techniques that work for a lot of men and women. And there are some likely pitfalls to avoid, unless you know your lover doesn't mind.

- Remove any jewelry from your hands that could get in the way, cause discomfort, or irritate your lover's genitals.
- Make sure your hands are clean.
- Use adequate lubrication at all times, whether you use saliva, oil, or commercial lubricant. Apply it regularly to maintain your lover's preferred balance of glide and friction.
- Change strokes occasionally. Mix it up and get creative. Variety is the spice of life. The element of surprise can help maintain excitement and keep your lover from losing the thread of arousal.

- Let yourself get turned on when giving your lover manual stimulation. Your arousal will feed your partner's arousal. If it doesn't distract you too much, you can even pleasure yourself at the same time.
- Allow your body to be in physical contact with your lover's. Press parts of your body into her. Let yourself dance as you play with her vulva.
- Use erotic talk or fantasy. Talk to your lover and tell her how much you desire her or weave a fantasy that is likely to assist in her arousal.
- Kiss your lover's mouth. Your mouth on your lover's can help him surrender even more to the pleasure you are providing.
- Stroke other parts of your lover's body with your free hand. Focus on areas you know are hot spots and likely to turn your lover on even more. Stimulating more than one erogenous zone at a time can really build the heat.

Feel the Connection

While manually pleasuring your lover, feel the connection between the two of you. This will greatly enhance the experience for both of you. It should never feel like a chore. Reconnect to the love you have for your partner. From time to time, look your lover in the eyes. Send her your love while witnessing her in her vulnerable state of ecstasy.

Bringing Him to Orgasm with Your Hand

Penises like to be touched. They present themselves in a way that let you know that—all out there in the open to be admired and appreciated. Most men have been touching themselves since they were young boys. Your male lover has most likely figured out how to touch himself in a way that feels good to him and brings him to orgasm. But having you take over will undoubtedly be a real treat, and it might be considerably more exciting for him.

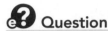 **Question**

How can I be sure to give him the kind of manual stimulation he likes?
Have your lover wrap his hand around yours, and start you off with both a pressure and a pace that feels good to him. At any time, he can bring his hand back to encourage you to apply different pressure or change the pace or rhythm.

The basic hand job involves using your palm and fingers to stroke up and down the shaft of his penis. Use a light or firm grasp, depending on his preference. And use lubrication to keep your hand from chaffing his skin. Start by keeping a steady pace or rhythm, unless he wants you to vary it. Let your stroke simulate what his penis might feel during penetration. Aim for smooth, gliding strokes. The pressure of your grip and the rhythm of the stroking can and should change over the course of your hand job.

Tips and Techniques

There is a lot of room for your own exploration in giving hand jobs. Try the following tips and techniques. Never forget that your lover is ultimately the expert. If it works for him, it's a good technique. If not, try another.

- Begin with feather-light, tickly movements using just the fingertips up and down the shaft of his penis. You can do this before you have applied any oil.
- Play with just the head of his penis. It is the most sensitive area. Lightly squeeze the coronal ridge with your fingertips. Circle around it and the frenulum with one finger, using feather-light upward strokes.

- If your male lover has some pre-cum secreting from the tip of his penis, you can use that to lubricate and titillate the head of his penis, before adding additional lube.
- Avoid the head of his penis for a while, as a way to tease your lover and help build the anticipation.
- Alternate hand over hand. Use only downward strokes from the head of his penis to the base. Lift each hand as it finishes its stroke, bringing it back to the head again, without stroking back up the shaft. If you rapidly alternate this stroke with both hands you can give him the sensation of an endless tunnel, or penetrative entry.
- Use a corkscrew motion to spiral your stroke down or up his penis.
- Use both hands together for stroking. This allows the penis to feel totally engulfed and can also make your man feel really big, so big that you have to use two hands to wrap all the way around him.
- Some men like to have their testicles lightly cupped or stimulated during a hand job. See what your man thinks about this.
- Use one hand to firmly grasp the base of his penis as the other hand strokes the shaft and the head. This can allow you to stroke very firmly and intensely without him feeling any uncomfortable tugging or pulling.
- Find your rhythm with each new stroke, getting into a groove. This will enable him to surrender more fully. Consistency can help establish an erotic trance and get him closer to orgasm.

Time for Orgasm and Ejaculation

When you are ready to bring your male lover to orgasm, increase the intensity and pace of your strokes. You might increase the pressure too, if that's okay with him. Be consistent with this higher-intensity stroking until he comes.

The head of your lover's penis may become very sensitive upon ejaculation, so ease up a bit as he completes his orgasm. Check with him to see what he prefers. When your lover ejaculates, you may choose to let him come on your hand, some other part of your body, his own body, or on a washcloth or towel. It helps to have a plan for this ahead of time.

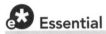 **Essential**

> Comment on how big and hard and beautiful your lover's penis is. Let him know how much it turns you on to be touching him, or how much you love giving him pleasure. These types of compliments and reassurances will help him surrender more to the experience.

After he orgasms, you can help him surrender to the pleasure he is experiencing. Rest one hand lightly over the shaft of his penis and the other over his heart. Just be present with him as he comes back to resting. This is a good time to share with your lover how much you love him or how beautiful he is, or to just enjoy peacefulness together.

Bringing Her to Orgasm with Your Hand

The skill of bringing your female lover to orgasm with your hand is likely to be very appreciated. Your fingers may be the most effective way to supply the direct clitoral stimulation many women require to achieve orgasm. Training your fingers exactly how to satisfy your lover, however, usually requires a willingness to both experiment and listen to feedback. Learning how she uses her fingers to masturbate is a good place to start. Unfortunately, not all women are comfortable with self-pleasuring, so she might have as much to learn as she has to teach about how to pleasure her.

You may need to try different things and ask her for feedback. Remember to be prepared for more peaks, plateaus, and dips with your female lover. It can be more of an up and down ride than with a man. There may be multiple starts and stops. Don't get discouraged. The end result will be worth all of the fuss.

 Alert

> The clitoral head has the most nerve endings and is the most sensitive part of the clitoris. That's why it feels so good to be touched, but it can be easily over-stimulated. Be careful not to over-focus on the head of the clitoris, unless she asks for that.

Tips and Techniques for Her

Your hand can stimulate her entire vulva, including her labia, clitoris, and the inside of her vagina, if she wants that. Don't limit yourself to just fingering the head of her clitoris. If you remember from the chapter on anatomy, the whole clitoris extends to just underneath the surface of the inner labia, where most of the erectile tissue of the clitoris lies. Stimulating the entire vulva allows for a larger area to become engorged, increasing arousal immensely for the woman, which will ultimately culminate in a richer, fuller, more satisfying orgasm. Here are some more tips and techniques that can help you give your female lover profound erotic pleasure with your hands:

- If your hands are too rough for the delicate tissue of her vulva, use a latex or vinyl glove with some lube.
- Be careful with your nails. The tissues of the genitals are very sensitive and can easily be aggravated by long, sharp, or jagged nails.
- The inside of your lover's vagina may supply adequate lubrication for a hand job. Dip a finger gently and slowly into the vagina to pull some of that wetness to her vulva. If not, just add some oil or lubricant.

- When fingering a woman, you can use the fingers of your free hand to spread open her outer labia, making the inner parts of her vulva more accessible.
- When stimulating the vulva, let your fingers glide smoothly over the clitoral hood and down both sides of the inner labia.
- Spread your touch around the vulva. Alternate between teasing the vaginal opening with light finger circling and stroking the clitoris.
- When stimulating the head and shaft of the clitoris, try different strokes and mix them up. Use just the tip of your forefinger or both your forefinger and middle finger. Use a circular motion or a figure-eight, or rub back and forth over the top of the head and shaft.
- You can also try lightly tapping the head and shaft with your fingertip. Or you can use a flickering motion with your finger.
- For extra fun and exploration, try gently gripping the shaft of the clitoris between your thumb and forefinger and stroke it up and down as if it was a very small penis. Feel it get harder and more engorged. Alternatively, you can lightly grip the clitoral shaft between your forefinger and middle finger, and twiddle your fingers back and forth.
- If and when she is ready to have the inside of her vagina stimulated, you can slide a finger or two inside of her. To start, just let them rest there while you continue to stimulate the rest of her vulva. Then begin to slide them in and out repeatedly. Make sure there is plenty of lubrication so that your fingers glide in smoothly and effortlessly. This is likely to heighten her arousal tremendously.
- Once she is really turned on, thrust your fingers along the front wall of the vagina (toward the stomach) where the famous G-spot is located. Try stroking her G-spot with a come-hither motion. She may or may not like this. Be sure

to check in with her about where she feels her G-spot and how she likes it touched.

All the Way to Orgasm

When your lover seems ready to orgasm, keep a steady, continual stroke on her clitoris. Be careful not to overdo the pressure, especially if you are feeling excited yourself. She may not want more pressure or a faster pace, just consistent stroking. If your lover does not want direct clitoral stimulation, let her tell you want she does want.

After she comes, her clitoris may become very sensitive, and she may want you to stop stimulating it. Your cooperation can help her enjoy the aftermath of her orgasm. Alternatively, she may want continued stimulation to help her have multiple orgasms. Again, let her feedback be your guide.

Once she has entirely completed her orgasm, rest one hand lightly over her entire vulva, and the other over her heart, allowing her to feel your presence still as her body comes back to resting. This is a good time to share any tender feelings you have for her, letting her know how beautiful she is to you, and how much you love her.

CHAPTER 10

Put Your Body Where My Mouth Is: Oral Paths to Orgasm

Using your mouth to stimulate your lover's genitals and other erogenous zones is another very gratifying way to help bring her to climax. The oral path to orgasm is a very intimate experience and can be incredibly stimulating for the giver as well. The sight, taste, smell and feel of your lover's body can be taken in like a smorgasbord of sensual delights. Meanwhile, the warm and wet sensation of your silky mouth on your lover's body is likely to make her sing out an orgasm like no other.

The Art of Oral Pleasure

Erotic pleasure, delivered via the mouth, is truly an art. Learning to use your mouth, including your lips, teeth, and tongue, to satisfy your lover will likely earn you many bonus points in your intimate relationships. Oral pleasure can be used either as foreplay or as the main path to orgasm. Because mouths are warm and wet, they provide tremendous sensation and ample lubrication to the stimulation you deliver this way. They seem to be designed perfectly for providing such pleasure. Add some simple technique to this perfect design and you can create an erotic experience for your lover that is out of this world.

Receiving Oral Pleasure

Not everyone is comfortable receiving oral pleasure. Concerns about how your genitals look, smell, or taste can get in the way of your enjoyment. You may also be preoccupied with whether your partner feels burdened by the task. The most direct way to deal with these concerns is to communicate your discomfort with your lover. He may be able to assure you that he loves doing this, that it turns him on, and that your genitals look, smell, and taste fine. Alternatively, you can take some deep breaths and remind yourself that your lover probably wouldn't be doing this if he didn't want to. The more you can relax and surrender to the pleasure, the more gratifying it will be, and the more likely you will experience orgasms this way.

 Essential

If worries about cleanliness or smells are getting in the way of enjoying oral pleasure, then bathe or shower beforehand. Consider, though, that your lover might really enjoy your unwashed taste and smell. Some lovers even like oral pleasure after a sweaty workout because of the smells produced and the taste of salt on the skin.

Giving Oral Pleasure

The mouth has many ways of delivering pleasure. You can be creative as you explore the many ways you can use your mouth to create enjoyable sensations for your lover. Try using your tongue in different ways. The variety can include full-blown kitty-cat licks with your whole tongue, making circles and figure eights, or flickering rapidly with just the tip. Play around with sucking, using your lips and teeth to create a vacuum. This can draw more blood to your partner's genitals and erogenous zones. Use your teeth by gently nibbling or more aggressively biting various parts of your lover's body. Breathe onto your lover's genitals or other erogenous zones, either by pressing your open mouth against her or by blowing air through your lips. You can mix and match all of these techniques, discovering whatever you and your lover enjoy.

Fellatio

Giving "head" or a "blow job" to a man can be quite fun. The clinical term for oral sex on a man is derived from the Latin word *fellatio*, meaning "to suck." Whatever you call it, the sensation of a warm and wet mouth wrapped around a man's penis is a unique and erotic experience like no other. The mouth can create so many different sensations that some men prefer oral stimulation of the penis to any other kind. To the giver of fellatio, the penis offers itself as a fascinating toy. When you play with it right, you make its owner squirm with pleasure.

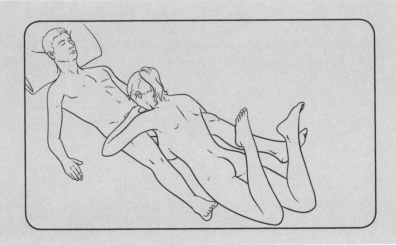

Starting Off

When performing fellatio on your male lover, it is important to find a position that you can both comfortably stay in for a while. When you take care of your own body's comfort, you are better able to provide for your partner. As you go along, you may want to shift positions from time to time to avoid any discomfort for either of you. Try sitting comfortably between his legs or at his side as he lies face up before you. Alternatively, lie down on your side with the side of your head resting on his pelvis. Or consider kneeling or squatting in front of him as he sits or stands. One of the benefits of performing fellatio is that you really don't need a bed for it. You can do it just about anywhere!

 Fact

The ancient Roman emperor Gallienus called fellatio *lesbiari*, because it was women from the island of Lesbos who were believed to have been the first to practice oral pleasure. In ancient Greece, fellatio was referred to as "playing the flute," and in the Kama Sutra, it is referred to as "mouth congress."

Tips and Techniques

When performing fellatio, there are many tips and techniques to keep in mind. Most importantly, have fun and enjoy the eroticism yourself. Imagine how good it would feel to have your lover inside of other parts of you with that erect penis of his. Enjoy how he surrenders to the pleasure and how turned on he is getting. Know that you are responsible. You can also begin anticipating the pleasures he may give you in return.

Use Your Hands

Your hands are valuable assistants during fellatio. You might even start off by stimulating his penis with your hands, adding your mouth later. You may want to use a hand on his penis the whole time. Your hands can help guide his penis where you want it to go, giving you more control than using just your mouth. Hand squeezes can also help give him the feeling of more engulfment, especially when they provide pressure at the base of his penis. Hand strokes can also keep up the stimulation whenever you need to give your jaw a break. They offer a way to add variety to the sensations you provide.

Licking the Whole Shaft and Head

Try licking the whole shaft and head of his penis as if it were a popsicle. Lick the head of his penis like it is the tastiest part. Use your whole tongue and go slow. Savor every lick. This will make his penis feel very loved and appreciated and help build the anticipation for your whole mouth to be on him.

 Alert

> Be careful with your teeth! The scariest thing for a man receiving fellatio is the threat of teeth accidentally clenching down on his delicate member. It is crucial that you find a way to keep your teeth clear of his penis. If you can demonstrate that you have this awareness, he will be able to surrender more to the pleasure.

Using Your Whole Mouth

There is nothing quite like the sensation of a wet, soft, and silky mouth sensually gliding up and down over a man's penis. Alternate between engulfing just the head for a while and then as much of the shaft as you can manage. It feels really good if you can engulf his whole penis with your mouth. Use your tongue in fun and creative ways to increase the sensations. You can also use one hand at the base of his penis while your mouth covers the rest to give him the sensation of total engulfment.

Deep Throating

If you are really adventurous, you can try deep throating, which refers to taking his penis all the way into your throat. Some men really like this. Deep throating requires that you relax the muscles in your throat and get past your gag reflex. It will help to relax and open up your throat if you can tilt your head back, so try this lying on your side, or with your head over the edge of the bed. You may want to practice on a dildo for starters.

Giving His Testicles Some Attention

Your male lover might like having his testicles stimulated during oral pleasure to his penis. You can try gently sucking on his testicles, or use a hand to lightly cup or stroke his testicles while your mouth is stimulating the head and shaft of his penis. It's a good idea to check in with him about the pressure on his testicles, since they can be very sensitive.

Stimulate His Other Erogenous Zones with Your Hands

When you have a free hand, use it to stimulate other erogenous zones on his body, such as his anus or perineum, his nipples, and his mouth and lips. Just make sure the additional stimulation is not distracting you or him from what you are doing with your mouth. It should contribute to the experience, not take away from it.

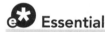 **Essential**

It is a good idea to plan ahead if you are going to be simulating your lover's P-spot. He should use the bathroom first to vacate his bladder and bowels. You should wash your hands and make sure there are no jagged edges on your nails. Also, you should have latex or vinyl gloves and lots of lubrication handy.

Stimulating the P-Spot

Men can get a lot of pleasure from the stimulation of their prostate gland or P-spot. As with a woman's G-spot, prostate stimulation can add greatly to a man's orgasmic experience when stimulated at just the right time. It usually feels best when he is already very turned on and close to orgasm. In order to access the P-spot, you will need to insert a finger, palm side up, about an inch into his anus. Make sure you use plenty of lube and that he is relaxed and ready. Once inside his anus, press your finger toward his navel. You are aiming to feel a round bulb of spongy tissue. When you find it, stroke the area with a come-hither motion and explore other ways to stimulate this area, checking in with him to see what he prefers.

Tease Him

Rather than bringing your lover to orgasm as fast as you can, why not tease him a bit? Bring him right up to the edge and then back off so that you can prolong the experience for him. This can help him build up more of a charge, potentially leading to a more powerful orgasm. You can do this in any of three ways. Try stopping the stimulation altogether, changing the stimulation, or slowing the stimulation down. Then, once his arousal has dipped a little, start up again. Try increasing the pace or finding a new rhythm.

Taking Him All the Way There

When you are ready to bring your lover to orgasm, keep your rhythm steady and constant. Pick up the pace and increase the pressure a little bit—or a lot, if he asks for that. Keep going until he comes. Decide ahead of time how you want to handle his semen as it ejaculates. If you do not want to get cum in your mouth, you can pull your mouth away and finish him off with your hand. Just make sure you do this in time. If you are using a condom, you won't have to worry about this.

If you let your lover come inside of your mouth, you have the choice of either swallowing his cum or spitting it out. It is certainly not harmful to swallow cum, but not everybody is comfortable doing that, for a variety of reasons. Your lover may really like it if you are willing to swallow his cum. It may help him feel more fully accepted. Many people find that they like the taste of cum and find it very satisfying to swallow. But don't feel bad if that is not your thing. If you need to, find a way to spit it out that won't make a big production of it.

Cunnilingus

There is nothing quite like the feeling of a warm, wet mouth on the vulva and clitoris. The tongue, with all of its flexibility and maneuvering abilities, has tremendous potential to give a woman erotic pleasure and bring her to orgasm. Some call it "going down," "eating out," or "giving head," but the clinical term for oral stimulation of the vulva or clitoris is *cunnilingus*. The word is derived from the Latin words "vulva" and "lick." Licking the vulva of your female lover is a classic way to really get her juices flowing.

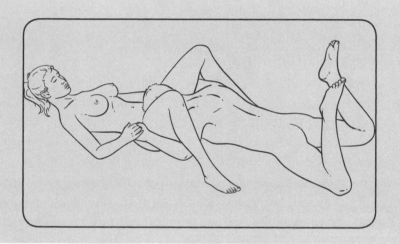

Starting Off

Start by getting into a position that is comfortable for you, especially if you have the intention of bringing your lover all the way to orgasm. You might be there for a while! Try lying face down on a flat surface with your head in between her legs. She should be lying face up with knees bent and feet planted on either side of you, or wrapped around your back. You may want to raise her hips with a pillow for her comfort or to lift her pelvis up higher for you. You may also place a pillow under your chest to support you. Another alternative position would be to have her sitting on a chair with her pelvis forward and her legs spread open. In this position she presents her vulva to you as you kneel before her. You can also try having her squat or kneel over your face as you lie down.

 Fact

According to Chinese Taoism, performing cunnilingus is way to increase one's vitality. The ingestion of vaginal fluids, or feminine elixir, is considered a health practice. Fellatio, on the other hand, is advised against, because of the threat of it leading to ejaculation, which in this tradition is believed to deplete a man's vitality.

Tips and Techniques

There are many ways to make cunnilingus really enjoyable for your lover. Above all, make sure she can relax into it. Women may be insecure about the taste or smell of their vulvas. Therefore, it is never a bad idea to let her know how much you love her taste and smell. Reassure her that you are happy to pleasure her. Let her know she can simply receive and enjoy. Then explore and discover the many ways to pleasure her with your mouth, paying attention to what works best for her. The following are some tips and techniques that should either get you off to a good start or take you to some new places.

 Alert

When giving oral pleasure to your lover, be sure to take care of your own body. Change your position as much as needed in order to stay comfortable. If your neck, shoulders, or jaw start to get uncomfortable, take a break. There is no need for one of you to suffer in order for the other to receive pleasure.

Use Your Hands

Your hands can be very instrumental when performing cunnilingus on your lover. You can start pleasuring her with your hands before putting your mouth on her. As a way to say hello, try lightly stroking her clitoris and labia. Your hands can also take over when your mouth and tongue get tired. Your fingers can be used for vaginal penetration, if and when she wants it.

Labia Licking

When bringing the tongue in on the action, try using your whole tongue with slow broad strokes along either side of her vulva. Go from the vaginal opening all the way up to the clitoris. Lick like you don't want to lose a single drop of her precious juices. Then, gradually start playing around with different kinds of strokes and pressure. Use different parts of your tongue. Have fun and enjoy the sensuousness of the labial tissues.

Focus on the Clitoris

At some point, you should begin to focus on her clitoris, unless direct stimulation of it is too intense for her. Try using firm solid pressure with your tongue and make slow, circular motions over the clitoral shaft and head. Gradually shift to figure-eight motions with your tongue. Then add variety by going side to side. You can also try sucking on her clitoris and see how she likes that. Continue to mix it up, but stay in a groove for a while with each new pattern your mouth finds. Ever so gradually, increase the pace. Be careful not to over-stimulate her clitoris with excessive speed or pressure.

Include Some Vaginal Penetration with Your Fingers

Many women want vaginal penetration to get really turned on or to orgasm. Check with your lover about this. If she gives you the thumbs up, start with one or two fingers. When she is ready, either lick your fingers with your own saliva, add other lubrication, or rely on her heavily flowing vaginal juices if she has them. Slowly and gently, insert your fingers, palm side up. Once your fingers are inside of her, just rest them there for a while, as you continue to lick and stimulate her vulva and clitoris. Then, gradually move your fingers slowly inward and outward of her vagina.

 Essential

When penetrating your lover's vagina with your fingers, start out slow and gentle. Get into a rhythm and gradually let it build in speed, intensity, and depth. Listen to her body. Let her hips tell you when they want to pick up the pace and increase the intensity. They will most likely start to rock and thrust as she becomes more excited.

Stimulating the G-Spot

Often, if you stimulate a woman's G-spot while performing cunnilingus, you will send her to the stars. This works best once she is already very aroused and close to orgasm. It can greatly intensify her orgasm. To reach the G-spot you will need to insert one or two fingers, palm side up, inside of her vagina. Press toward her pubic bone, about one and a half to three inches in. You are feeling for a spongy bulb of tissue. When you find it, use a come-hither motion. Check in with your lover and explore any other motions that feel particularly good to her.

Stimulate Her Other Erogenous Zones with Your Hands

Use your free hand to stimulate her other erogenous zones—the ones you can reach from your perch at her vulva. You may caress the skin of her whole body, stimulate her breasts and nipples, or touch her lips and mouth. If she likes, you can stimulate her anus or perineum with a finger. Just make sure that the added stimulation is not too distracting for you or her. The manual stimulation should add to what you are doing with your mouth on her vulva, not take over the show.

Taking Her All the Way There

Bringing your female lover all the way to orgasm may require that you have both patience and endurance. Her arousal has to build at its own pace. It will help if the erotic energy between the two of you has been building for a while before starting cunnilingus. When you feel like she is getting closer, keep up the stimulation in a constant and steady manner. Be careful in your excitement not to overdo the pressure on her clitoris. It is fine to increase the pace a little bit, but let it build gradually. When she starts to come, don't back off of the stimulation just yet. See her all the way through the end of her orgasm, or until she asks you to stop.

 Fact

The enjoyment of cunnilingus is nothing new, evidence of the practice dates back as early as 300 B.C. Explicit depictions of cunnilingus have been found on ancient pottery from the tribal societies of Oceana, on ancient scrolls from China and Japan, and in ancient Indian temple carvings.

Once your lover has an orgasm, you may need to ease off of her clitoris, which will most likely be very sensitive at this point. Rather than abandoning her vulva altogether, however, you can cup your hand lightly over the entire area. This is a soft way to stay in contact with her as she makes her descent back down to resting. It allows the two of you to bask in the afterglow of her orgasm.

Variations of Oral Pleasure

There are many more ways to give and receive oral pleasure. If you feel adventuresome and are ready to explore new territory, read on. Whether you get really turned on using your mouth on your lover's body or you just love what it does for her, the following variations offer some interesting new routes to orgasm.

Simultaneous Oral Pleasure

Giving and receiving oral pleasure simultaneously, often referred to as the 69 position, is another way to enjoy oral sex. To try it, have your lover lie on his back with his knees up or down. Then, facing his feet, crouch down on all fours over your lover's head and lower your genitals to your lover's mouth. At the same time lower your face to your lover's genitals. You may find that giving and receiving simultaneously is a highly erotic way to build excitement between you and your lover. You can also try a variant of this position where you and your partner both lie on your sides.

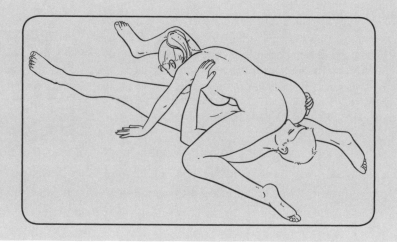

Oral-Anal Stimulation

Oral-anal stimulation, also called analingus or "rimming," involves using your tongue or mouth to stimulate your lover's anus. While this is certainly not for everyone, the tissue of the anus is full of nerves and therefore very sensitive. Thus, analingus may be highly erotic for many people.

 Alert

> There are many diseases that you need to be concerned about if you engage in analingus. These include Hepatitis A, E. coli, intestinal parasites, bacterial infections, gonorrhea, syphilis, and herpes. It is, therefore, very important to take adequate precaution when engaging in oral-anal stimulation. In contrast, the risk of contracting HIV through analingus is very low.

If you would like to try it, be sure to take note of health precautions. At the very least, make sure that your lover has thoroughly washed his anus and that there is no fecal matter present before you use your lips or tongue on him. To be extra safe, use plastic wrap, a dental dam, or a ripped up condom between his anus and your mouth. This will help protect you from the various diseases you could possibly contract.

Once you have taken all adequate precautions, you can explore the tissue of your lover's anus with your tongue and mouth. Try encircling the rim of the anus with your tongue, licking side to side and even penetrating the anus as much as he likes and as much as you feel comfortable doing. You can also stimulate the area just between the anus and the genitals, called the perineum, which is also full of nerves and therefore very sensitive.

Oral Pleasure to Other Erogenous Zones

Your lover's genitals are not the only parts of her body that are capable of deriving erotic pleasure from your mouth. See what other parts might be responsive. Take a tour of your lover's whole body with your lips, tongue, teeth, and open mouth. Lick, suck, nibble, bite, and blow your way around her magnificent landscape. See the different responses you get from the toes and fingers, ears, neck, nipples, and navel.

Getting Creative with Your Oral Pleasure

One way to get creative and have a little more fun with oral sex is to add some delicious flavors or treats. Stimulating your taste buds can make your sexual experience even more sensual. One option is to purchase flavored lubricants or condoms. Or you can try kissing and passing candy, mints, or gum back and forth between your mouths. Another option is to use syrup or liqueurs. Pour them on each other's genitals and lick them off. Try smearing food on each other's erogenous zones and then devour each other. Certain flavors like mint or cinnamon can add a tingly sensation—especially noticeable on the genitals—that your lover may really get into.

 Essential

When exploring your lover's various erogenous zones with your mouth, you may find a responsive body part. She may communicate this to you verbally with her moans and other sounds of delight or with her body movements. When you find a responsive spot, hang out there for a while. See how much pleasure she can handle in that one area before you move on to another.

Yet another way to get creative is to play with the temperature and sensation. Try using an ice cube in your mouth as you give oral pleasure to your lover's genitals or other erogenous zones. Sometimes cooling things down can really heat things up! Or warm your mouth with some hot water or tea before performing cunnilingus or fellatio. See how the extra heat adds to your partner's pleasure.

CHAPTER 11

Penetration and Orgasms

There is nothing quite like the powerful sensation of penetrating or being penetrated. For most people, this is the pinnacle of excitement and sexual expression with a lover, and what many people consider as the most intimate you can be with another person. The path to orgasm through penetration is therefore often given the most recognition and status of all the sexual behaviors. Regardless of how penetration currently ranks in your book, this route offers tremendous possibility to deepen your experience of orgasm and take your pleasure to new heights.

The Act of Penetration

Penetration feels good, but it could be said that the urge to penetrate or be penetrated stems from the desire to energetically merge with another. Many people feel penetration gives you a sense of closeness that you don't get from other sex acts, which can emotionally intensify the experience of orgasm. And, of course, being penetrated allows for certain internal parts that would otherwise go untouched to be stimulated, creating what many consider to be a much fuller, richer, and more satisfying physical experience. For many men, the act of penetration is the preferred route to orgasm. Women, on the other hand, are not as inclined to orgasm through penetration alone, and therefore penetration ranks lower for many women as a preferred path to orgasm. However, women who manage to receive clitoral stimulation and thus achieve orgasm during penetration rate their experience of penetration much higher.

The Various Forms of Penetration

Penetrating and being penetrated can happen in a variety of ways, with a variety of implements. In this day and age, you can't just assume that when someone refers to penetration, they are referring to penis-vagina intercourse. There are many ways in which people like to penetrate and be penetrated, and some relationships allow for certain kinds of penetration and not others. Two men together naturally can't have vaginal intercourse, but they can have anal intercourse or anal penetration with an object. Two women can't have penis-vagina intercourse, but they can engage in intercourse with a dildo or penetration with an object. If a man wants to receive anal penetration from his female lover, she can use a strap-on dildo to penetrate him anally—this is known as "pegging." A couple in which the man has difficulty with an erection may choose to use an object for penetration. These are just a few scenarios that call for varied forms of penetration.

Vaginal Penetration

Vaginal penetration can happen in several ways—with a penis, with the use of another body part, or with the use of an object. While all of these involve stimulating the vagina, each has the potential to create very unique sensations and overall experiences. In general, women who like penetration like the feeling of having their vaginas filled. They like the pressure that is created from having something inside of them. A woman's preferred kind of vaginal penetration could be based on a variety of factors, including past experiences, relationship choices, and her body's response to the sensations created by the different forms of penetration.

Intercourse can refer to penetration of the vagina with a penis or with a strap-on dildo. Penis-vagina intercourse requires, of course, a biological man and a biological woman. It is the only procreative sex and what many people think of when they hear the word "sex." However, it is more than just a path to procreation, and it is only one of many paths to orgasm. For many, penis-vagina intercourse is truly the primary route to ecstasy. With penis-vagina intercourse, both parties are simultaneously genitally stimulated, and the pleasure is shared, which has certain advantages and disadvantages.

 Fact

Intercourse can also refer to penetration with a strap-on dildo. Although the dildo itself does not experience any stimulation, the person wearing it can get turned on and stimulated enough to achieve orgasm, aided by various attachments, and by her own bumping and grinding motion that can stimulate the clitoris.

Using a body part, such as fingers, known as "digital penetration," or a whole hand, known as "fisting," to penetrate the vagina, is another option. Some women prefer the use of fingers to stimulate the inside of their vagina because of the dexterity of fingers and their ability to focus or direct their stimulation on the G-spot in just the right way. Using the whole hand can give a woman a sense of really being filled vaginally, which is highly erotic and pleasurable for some women. When your lover is using her fingers or hand to penetrate you, the primary focus is your pleasure, which can render some amazing orgasms.

Some women find the use of objects, such as dildos, to be just the right thing to penetrate them. There are many objects that can provide wonderful stimulation for the vagina, which will be discussed in depth in Chapter 12. Again, when using an object for penetration, the focus is all on the recipient's pleasure, giving her a feeling of being catered to or pampered.

Anal Penetration

Anal penetration, like vaginal penetration, can happen in several ways—with a penis, other body parts such as fingers or the whole hand, or with an object such as a butt plug or dildo. More and more people are discovering the pleasures of anal penetration and intercourse. Once a highly taboo sexual activity, anal stimulation is now becoming more accepted and mainstream. While it is still an activity that makes a lot of people squirm with discomfort, many bold and curious pioneers are setting out to discover this new frontier of pleasure for themselves.

For some people, anal sex is erotic partially because of its taboo status, but for others it is erotic solely because of the sensations that are created when the anus is stimulated. The anus has many nerve endings that can create tremendous arousal when stimulated. For men, anal sex stimulates the prostate gland, or the P-spot, which is the male version of the G-spot.

The main things to keep in mind with any kind of anal play are adequate lubrication and relaxation of the anal sphincter muscle. You will need a tremendous amount of lube when engaging in anal intercourse or penetration. This is because the rectum and anus do not have any natural lubrication, and the tissue is very sensitive and vulnerable to tearing and soreness. Also, because the anal sphincter muscle is very strong, you will need to spend a fair amount of time focusing on relaxing it. This can take a fair amount of patience.

 Alert

Safety is a real concern with anal intercourse in particular. The tissues of the anus and rectum are very delicate and tear easily, making the presence of blood more likely, and therefore infection more probable. Make sure that you know the risks involved and take necessary precautions. To stay on the safe side, always use condoms.

Who's in Charge?

Because of the inherent vulnerability of being penetrated, the one who is being penetrated is ultimately in charge. In other words, you take responsibility for what feels good to you, and communicate with your lover how to direct the penetration so that it adds to your pleasure and arousal and does not cause any discomfort or pain. This is particularly important to remember when engaging in forms of penetration that involve a penis. That is because the person penetrating is also being genitally stimulated, and may therefore be distracted by, and focusing on, his own pleasure so much so that he loses his awareness of your experience.

Active or Passive?

In nearly every position with any kind of penetration, it is possible for either or both partners to be the active one, although it is typically the person who is providing the penetration. Being the active partner requires more work, but it has the benefit of allowing you to be in control of the movement in a way that satisfies you. You can give yourself the angle and the depth of penetration that feels good to you. Because one needs to be fairly relaxed in order to open and receive penetration, it is usually the recipient of penetration who is the passive partner. But some people like to be active as they are being penetrated, at least some of the time. Regardless of what your preference is for being active or passive during penetration, there are benefits to sharing that role. You can give the active partner a break and you can also demonstrate how you like penetration, showing your partner what feels good to you.

Readiness for Penetration

The most important question to ask before engaging in penetration each and every time is whether or not each person is ready. Penetration is a particularly vulnerable act, and it is thus very important to take extra precaution in making sure you are both in the right place for it. There are both physiological and psychological factors that play into being ready for penetration. Overlooking any of these factors could be detrimental to yourself or your relationship with your lover. Knowing how to assess your own readiness, as well as your lover's, could help you avoid any potential harm or damage to yourself, your lover, or the relationship. Everyone has her own preconditions for penetration, but here are some likely candidates for conditions that need to be met in order for you to be interested and ready to go.

Is the Relationship Where You Need It To Be?

How you are feeling toward your lover factors into whether you want to engage in penetration with her, as well as the quality of the connection when you do. Generally speaking, it is good if you both feel close and connected, and not angry or resentful. Sometimes couples use sex to feel closer and more connected to each other, and if this works for you—great! But having sex when you are angry or feeling resentful is potentially very harmful to your connection and could taint your feelings pertaining to the act of intercourse for one or both of you.

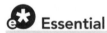 **Essential**

Before engaging in penetration, you and your partner should both feel your relationship is loving, trusting, and safe. This will help with the quality of the connection and will most likely influence your overall feelings about penetration in the long run. The more you both enjoy it now, the more you are both likely to want to engage in it in the future.

Is It a Good Time?

So many factors can play into whether or not it is a good time to engage in penetration, but the most important are whether there is enough time for it to be satisfying for the both of you, and whether you will be able to be present for the experience. While there is certainly nothing wrong with a "quickie," you want to be sure that there is sufficient time for everyone who wants an orgasm to have one and that you can both enjoy the encounter. If you need to be somewhere or get some sleep, or if your mind is occupied with all the things you need to get done, then you will probably not be able to show up for the encounter in a way that is mutually satisfying for both of you. You will be better off waiting until the time is right. If the time is always right for intercourse for you and your lover, then you should both count your blessings.

Are You Adequately Turned On?

When engaging in anal or vaginal intercourse, it is essential that both parties be adequately turned on in order for the experience to feel good to both of you. There is a particular a danger with intercourse in which the one being penetrated may not be as aroused as the person penetrating. This is something to look out for. If this is a dynamic that pervades in your relationship for any length of time, then your sexual relationship is at risk of coming to a stand-still somewhere in the future. Better tend to it now, before your partner decides she just doesn't like, want, or need penetration, period.

It is also possible for a man to put pressure on himself or feel pressure from his partner to engage in penetration and perform in a way that he doesn't feel ready to do, emotionally or physiologically. Contrary to some people's beliefs, men have preconditions for engaging in sex and are not always up for the task.

Ready to Receive Vaginal Penetration?

Although every vagina is unique, it generally takes a while for a vagina to be ready for penetration. Vaginas often need considerable foreplay and teasing before they are ready to be penetrated. If you are a woman, being adequately turned on for intercourse or penetration with an object means there is some natural lubrication and engorgement of the tissues of your vulva and vagina. The more turned on and aroused you are, the better the penetration will feel to you. Regardless of what is being used to penetrate your lover's vagina, keep this in mind: Pamper the vulva, and especially the clitoris, before moving into any form of penetration.

> **EXERCISE:** The next time you are the recipient of vaginal penetration with a partner, see how aroused you can get before you engage in penetration. You should be so turned on that you feel some pulsing in your vagina, and a deep yearning to be entered. Your pelvis may even start rocking and looking for the action.

Ready to Receive Anal Penetration?

Being ready for anal penetration requires that you be relaxed. Your anus, especially, will need to be relaxed enough to enjoy the sensation of penetration. The anus often needs a fair amount of teasing and playing lightly around its opening before it is ready to open more. Never force anal penetration. Take your time and let the anus gradually open to the penetration. Take lots of deep breaths and focus on relaxing the tissues around your anus. Start small and work up to more. The more you engage in anal play, the more the anus will learn how to relax enough to receive penetration.

So Many Positions, So Little Time

There are many more possible positions for penetration than most people venture to explore. You may have found a position that works for you and basically gets the job done. Hopefully this position works for your lover too! But why stop there? There are many reasons to explore new positions, including the following:

- Trying new positions can help get you out of a rut in your sex life.
- Exploring alternative positions may put you more into your body.

- You may discover new sensations because of the angles that different positions offer.
- You may find a position that significantly increases your arousal.
- You might discover a position that increases the likelihood of, or improves the experience of, your orgasms.

Whether you are engaging in a mutually stimulating form of penetration or a form in which only one of you is being stimulated, you can potentially find yourselves in any number of positions. The more free you feel in your body to explore different positions, the more likely you are to discover positions that really work for you. The following are some common positions for penetration, including some variations you can try. But don't stop there! Get creative and see if you can come up with some of your own.

Missionary Position

The missionary position is by far the most common position for intercourse used around the world. This position can also be used for anal intercourse. In this position, the person being penetrated lies face up, and the one penetrating lies face down on top of the other. There are many variations of this, mostly related to how the person on the bottom places her legs. You can have your knees bent with your feet flat on the ground on either side of your male lover. Or your knees can be bent, legs separated and lifted into the air, or wrapped around your lover. Or one or both of your legs can lift on or over his shoulders or arms. The one penetrating can support himself with his arms, giving whatever amount of his weight works for you both.

The missionary position has the benefit of possible eye contact and the feeling of your vulnerable underbellies exposed to each other. In this position, you can also appreciate the visual of each other's faces and the front of your bodies. The one penetrating generally feels like he has a lot of control in this position to thrust and move his hips, enabling him to get the kind of penetration and stimulation that works best for him to achieve orgasm. If you like to be a passive recipient during penetration, the missionary position may work great for you. However, as the recipient, you can also rock and move your pelvis in a way that allows you to have some control of the stimulation being provided.

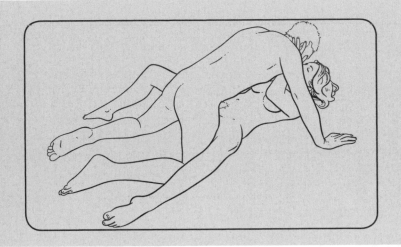

Play around with the variations at different stages of arousal to see what works when. As the person being penetrated gets more turned on and closer to orgasm, she will often want deeper penetration. For this, she may like the variation where her legs are up over her lover's shoulders or arms, which both tilts her pelvis at a nice angle and gives his penis greater accessibility to her vagina or anus.

Female-on-Top Positions

Female-on-top positions for intercourse are those in which—you guessed it—the woman is on top. Of course, these positions could also be used for a man receiving anal penetration. The partner doing the penetrating lies face up. There are many ways for the recipient of penetration to position herself. She can lie on top, face up or down, straddle her lover with legs straight out on either side of his torso, or with knees bent and feet flat on either side of him in a squatting position. She can also rest on her shins in a kneeling position, facing either toward his head or feet.

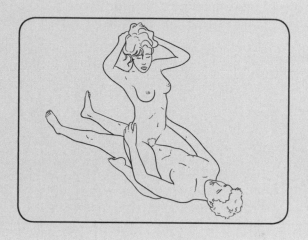

 Alert

In the recipient-on-top position, it is very important to watch how you angle your pelvis when your lover's penis is inside you. There are certain angles that are challenging for some erect penises. Be sensitive toward your lover's penis and check with him to see what angles work and don't work.

There are many benefits of this position, particularly for certain variations. The recipient has more control over movement, and women have easy clitoral access. Both partners can gaze at each other, and hands are free for stroking each other's other erogenous zones. Women who like a lot of breast and nipple stimulation can benefit greatly from the variation in which she squats or kneels on top facing her lover. Also, the recipient does not actually have to be active in this position. She can be passive and allow her lover to move his pelvis underneath her.

Rear-Entry Positions

Rear-entry positions are those in which the penetration comes from behind. These positions are very versatile and can be easily adapted to many forms of penetration. Whether you are lying face down on top of one another, on all fours while he kneels behind you, or both standing, this position offers an angle for penetration that really works for many people. You may find this position feels very natural and helps you get in touch with your animal essence. This position also lends itself well to the fantasy of taking—or being taken by—your lover.

Side-Lying Positions

Side-lying positions are those in which one or both of you are lying, in some shape or form, on your side. You can face each other or face the same direction in a rear entry position. He can be on his side facing you, while you lie on your back and out to the side, forming a T-shape and scissoring your legs with his, one leg between his and the other over his hips. These variations can give you a break from more strenuous positions, give you some new angle or penetration possibilities, and can be great for clitoral and other erogenous zone stimulation.

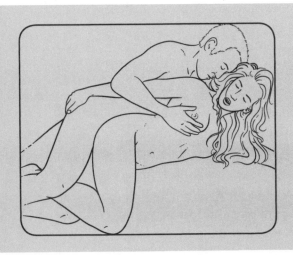

Seated Positions

Seated positions for intercourse generally work only with the woman sitting on top of the man. They can be done in a chair, on a couch, in a bed, or on the floor. You can face each other or face the same direction in a rear-entry position. If you are facing each other in a chair without arms, she can dangle her legs off to the sides. If you are facing the same direction, he will probably need to slide forward on the chair a bit, and/or she will need to lean forward a little, in order for the position and angle of the penis to work.

Yab yum, Tibetan for "father-mother," refers to a seated position often used in Tantra. In yab yum, the male sits in a cross-legged position, and the female sits on top of him, facing him, also cross-legged, wrapping her legs around him. These positions can provide very good depth of penetration, interesting angles to play with, and a lot of skin-to-skin contact that can feel particularly delightful and intimate. It can be harder, however, to apply certain penetration techniques, given the limited range of motion the hips are capable of in these positions.

Standing Positions

Standing positions are those in which one or both of you have your feet on the floor and are in an upright, vertical stance. They can be challenging, especially if you get weak in the knees, but they can also be tremendously fun and highly arousing. In order for this to be physically possible, your heights will have to be compatible, or one or both of you will need to be particularly acrobatic. Standing positions include both of you standing and facing each other, while he lifts one of your legs,

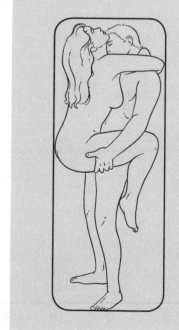

or you wrap it around him. You can stand and lift her up as she wraps both of her legs around you, or you can stand on the floor and bend over a table as he enters you from behind.

The Entry

The penetrative entry, regardless of who is penetrating whom, is something to pay attention to. Be present with the experience, for the sake of sensation and the emotional and energetic connection. Regardless of who is the active partner at the time of entry, that lover should move slowly and thoughtfully, thus creating feelings of emotional safety and trust.

Vaginal Penetration

With penis-vagina intercourse, moving slowly allows you both to fully experience the exquisite moment when your aroused genitals finally come into contact and begin to merge. Let this be a polite dance between your genitals, in which they are listening to each other intently to all the delightful and subtle pulsing and quivering that is going on. You both should sense that the vagina is very much inviting the penis in, rather than the penis just forcing its way in, or the vagina forcing its way around. The same should be true when using an object for vaginal penetration. The vagina should be inviting the object in.

Anal Penetration and Intercourse

To prepare for anal entry, you will want to take plenty of time relaxing your anal sphincter muscle. You can start this process by using lots of lube, playing around the rim for a good deal of time, and then slowly and gradually inserting one finger into the anus. It can help if you bear down and push the anal sphincter muscle out while you insert the finger.

Being ready for anal intercourse can take some time, and it requires a lot of patience initially. The muscles will eventually figure out how to relax more readily. The entry for any anal penetration should always be very slow and cautious and involve ample amounts of lubrication.

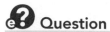 **Question**

How do I prepare myself for anal intercourse?
Start with one well-lubricated finger—preferably your own. Leave the finger in as long as you can and try and relax the anal sphincter muscles. Gradually work up to two and maybe three fingers. You may also prefer to use butt plugs, which come in many shapes and sizes.

Tips and Techniques for Penetration

Penetration is often rife with forceful and passionate thrusting that seems to come from a very primal place. This penetrative thrusting can overcome you and seem to have its own sense of purpose and mission that you may or may not agree with. It can take some time to learn how to handle or how to direct this force. But for the sake of more exquisite and refined pleasures, it is a force worth reckoning with. Here are some tips and techniques to keep in mind when engaging in penetration of any kind.

Take It Slow

Any penetration should always start out slow, unless your lover indicates that she wants something else. In order for the tissues of the vulva and vagina to relax and become aroused and engorged, they need to feel safe. Slow, careful movements will support a sense of safety for her. You can gradually build up the intensity of penetration, including the speed, depth, and force, always checking in with her to make sure it's working.

Use Lube When Necessary

Penetration often requires added lubrication. If a woman is ovulating or produces a lot of vaginal lubrication, you may not need to add any lube for vaginal intercourse, or even for vaginal penetration with an object. But for any anal play, count on needing a lot of lube. The penis or object that is penetrating the anus or vagina should feel as though it can glide inward and outward, effortlessly and smoothly, without causing any discomfort or pain.

Feel-Good Moves

Learning how to make penetration as delightful as possible requires some practice, exploration, and finesse. You may have already explored a wide range of movements for penetration and discovered some very gratifying moves for you and your lover. But, just in case you haven't yet caught on to these moves or have forgotten about them, here are a few tried and true methods.

Just the Tip

Penetrating with or engulfing just the tip of the penis (or object) is a wonderful sensation for both of you. This is a great way to start penetration, or to occasionally revisit during a lovemaking encounter. Using just the tip is a way to tease and build arousal, as well as increase lubrication before further penetration or engulfment. You can explore this with slow or quick movements, and everything in between. Try different angles and positions to find out how this feels best to both of you.

Taking Your Time

Gradually working your way to full penetration is a much more skillful and exciting way to approach penetration. This can help increase the sexual tension, get your energies and emotions more in touch with each other, and create a circumstance in which you can delight in the subtleties of sensation. Going slow also creates a sense of safety, which helps immensely with arousal and lubrication for women, providing a much more luscious experience for you both. If you have the urge to hurry things up, try taking some deep breaths, breathing in the pleasurable sensations you are experiencing in that moment.

 Fact

Stimulating the G-spot in women during vaginal penetration, or the P-spot in men during anal penetration, can greatly intensify the orgasmic experience. Aim for this spot during penetration, particularly as your lover gets close to orgasm. It could be the one trick that sends your lover over the edge.

Long, Slow, and Deep

Long, slow, and deep penetration is a great way to slow time, increase the size of your penis and increase arousal. After having gradually worked your way to full penetration, take some time just enjoying the lusciousness of the entire penis moving in and out of the vagina. Going slow can also create more space to fully recognize your feelings and enjoy your intimate connection with your lover.

All You've Got

When your passion peaks, giving all you've got and moving fast and forcefully can be just the thing to send you both over the edge, emotionally and physiologically. Wait until you absolutely can't hold back anymore and make sure that your lover is on the same page. You want to let the passion inside of you and between you and your lover build naturally, rather than forcing your movements.

The Afterglow

Penetration and the orgasms that are produced this way can put you into a very raw and vulnerable state. You may even be moved to tears. Often, a sense of deep connection and intimacy forms and can make you feel very tender toward your lover. You may be feeling that your energies have merged and that you are truly not alone. This is a wonderful time to indulge yourselves in feelings of closeness to each other.

 Essential

When your lover is ready to come, she may or may not want the penetration to continue. She may want it to stop so that she can focus on relaxing into the sensations and ride the pulsations and waves without the distraction of thrusting. Or she may want you to keep up the rhythm and groove until she has finished coming.

Is Everybody Coming?

Although it is not absolutely necessary for everyone to orgasm each time you engage in penetration, the more both of you come from this activity, the more appeal it will have and the more likely it is to happen with some regularity. If you are in a pattern in which only one of you comes during anal or vaginal intercourse, you will want to remedy this so that you both will continue to want to engage in these behaviors.

It is probably not a mystery to you that men are more likely to achieve orgasm during intercourse than women, but it doesn't have to be that way. In fact, given that women are more easily multi-orgasmic than men, women could potentially have more orgasms from intercourse than men. But in order for a woman to be orgasmic with intercourse, there are many things that you may both need to pay attention to.

Pay Attention to Her Arousal

Many women can lose the thread of arousal during intercourse. There are many reasons for this and just as many solutions. It can be helpful to check in with your female lover during intercourse to make sure it's still working for her, especially when you are getting the feeling that something is wrong. If she gets really quiet or motionless, this may be an indication that she is not into it, so it is worth checking in with her. It is easy to get lost in your own ecstasy and forget that there are two of you on this journey together, but it is highly beneficial to make sure you are both getting your needs met. Here are some things that a woman may need in order to catch the thread of arousal:

- Look into each other's eyes and feel the emotional connection
- Slow down the pace
- Add more lubrication
- Change position
- Change the angle or depth of penetration
- Switch to another sexual activity

 Alert

If something is not working for you as the recipient of anal or vaginal intercourse, then speak up. Chances are your lover would rather stop then and there and take care of your needs than do harm to you or the relationship. Don't be a martyr and think you need to endure painful penetration for the sake of your lover's pleasure.

Stimulate Her Clitoris

Most women do not get enough clitoral stimulation to achieve orgasm during intercourse. Remember, the clitoris is a woman's main route to orgasm, not her vagina, although the two together make a very powerful team for many women. It may be necessary for one or both of you to stimulate the clitoris at some point during intercourse. It doesn't necessarily have to be all the way through; you can find what works best by exploring different types of clitoral stimulation at different times.

Hold Off on Yours to Wait for Hers

If you are able to postpone your orgasm until your female lover comes, you will experience significant payoff by way of her future interest in this activity with you. You will need to learn how to cool your jets and recognize when you are at the edge so that you can pull back just in time. You too will benefit by prolonging your enjoyment of penetration with your lover.

CHAPTER 12

The Use of Sex Aids

People are capable of astounding creativity, especially when it comes to sex; many tools and toys have been invented to enhance erotic pleasure. A sex aid is any object or medium that is used to help increase sexual arousal, facilitate sex, or achieve an orgasm. There are many such products available for purchase. But an item does not have to be packaged and sold to be a sex aid. It can be a piece of furniture, something lying around your house, or some food in your refrigerator.

Lubricants

Lubricants are probably the single most commonly used sex aid. Natural vaginal lubrication is not always sufficient to make sex easy and comfortable, and the rectum does not produce any of its own lubrication. Lubricants are thus helpful in reducing friction in the vagina or anus during sexual play. Whether you are self-pleasuring, using sex toys, manually stimulating each other, or having intercourse, you will want to have plenty of lube available to keep things juicy!

Oils

Natural vegetable oils can feel wonderful when used in different kinds of erotic play. Coconut oil is an excellent choice because it is a little thicker than most. It also is easier to wash out of sheets than other oils. The main problem with vegetable oils is that contact with them can weaken latex. Thus, oil-based lubricants (vegetable or petroleum) should not be used with most condoms or any latex sex toy. Natural oils are not a problem, however, when used with vinyl condoms. Synthetic oil-based lubes, such as petroleum jelly, are generally not recommended. They, too, will break down latex and they tend to linger in the vagina or anus. This can be uncomfortable as well as make infection more likely to occur. There are much better alternatives as far as texture and consistency.

 Alert

Women should avoid using creams, lotions, or scented oils in the vagina. Many of these products irritate the vagina and can trigger yeast infections. Coconut oil, on the other hand, is considered by some to be a cure for yeast infections, and may help prevent them from occurring in the first place.

Water-Based Lubricants

Water-based lubes are the most popular and most-often recommended personal lubricants. They are made to be non-staining, non-irritating, and safe to use with all condoms. They are considered all-purpose lubes, meaning they are good for any sexual activity, with or without toys. They come in different consistencies, from liquid to jelly. Liquid lubes tend to have a consistency closest to saliva or your natural juices, so if you want something relatively light, go with these.

Jelly lubes are thicker and last longer. For anal sex or more extended encounters, you should go with them. Most water-based lubes are taste-free, except for the special flavored varieties made for oral sex. Water-based lubes are easy to wash off your person, your toys, or your bed sheets. Simply use soap and water.

Silicone-Based Lubricants

Silicone-based lubes are the slipperiest and longest lasting of the personal lubricants. They are handy for sex where there is water involved (in a bath or pool) because they will not rinse away. You do need to be careful when using them in the bathtub or shower because they can make surfaces very slippery. Silicone-based lubes are compatible with latex but are not recommended for use with condoms. If a silicone-based lube gets too dry, it may get sticky and the resulting friction can cause a condom to break. Also, using silicone-based lube with your silicone sex toys is not recommended, because they can degrade the texture of the silicone on your toy.

Sex Toys: Dildos, Vibrators, and More

Any object you use to help with sexual arousal and orgasm could be considered a sex toy. It can be a product designed for sexual use or it could be an object (like a cucumber) that you have adopted for use during sex. Sex toys are usually used to stimulate the genitals in some way. They can be used for self-pleasuring or for encounters with a lover.

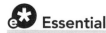 Essential

When choosing a sex toy, don't be fooled by looks. What is important is how an object functions and feels. Remember, no toy is going to feel like the real thing, even if it looks like the real thing. You may want to ask around and see what your friends have to say.

There are a plethora of sex toys on the market, and buying them is easier than ever. You can go online and shop discreetly from home. Or you can visit a specialty store that allows you to see, touch, and feel the toys up close and personal. It can be very helpful to get assistance from knowledgeable staff and have any of your burning questions answered. Choosing a sex toy can be challenging. You can't try them out beforehand, and once you buy one, you usually can't return it. You have to make a leap of faith as to what might feel good to you.

Dildos

Dildos are objects used for vaginal or anal penetration. They are more or less shaped like a penis—long and cylindrical—but vary to some degree in shapes and sizes. Some are completely

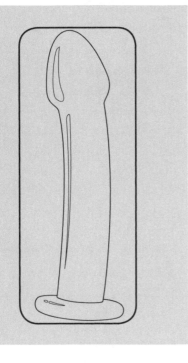

straight and some are curved. Some are completely smooth, while others have ridges and bumps. Some are made to look like real penises with glans, coronal ridge, veins, and all. You can find soft packs, dildos that are not completely firm, and dildos that come complete with testicles. Some dildos are designed specifically for G-Spot or prostate stimulation. You can get double-penetrators, made to penetrate both the vagina and anus simultaneously. "Double-enders" are dildos made to penetrate two people simultaneously. There are even inflatable dildos that allow you to get just the right size and firmness.

Dildos are made in a variety of different colors, materials, and textures. Dildos made from porous materials such as latex, jelly, and cyber-skin can be very soft. They need to be kept extra clean, however, because bacteria and viruses can live in the small holes on the surface. Also, when using porous dildos, you will need to apply lubrication regularly because the pores will absorb the lubrication. Dildos made from non-porous materials such as silicone, acrylic, vinyl, glass, or metal can also be very smooth. They will need less lubrication and will not harbor viruses or bacteria, but they still need to be kept clean.

When choosing a dildo, here are some questions to consider:

- How much are you willing to spend?
- Do you have a latex allergy or sensitivity to any other materials?
- What texture seems appealing?
- Will you be using the dildo anally or vaginally?
- Do you want something that can stimulate your G-spot or P-spot?
- Do you think you would like simultaneous anal and vaginal penetration?
- Do you want to use this toy with a partner? How?
- Do you want something that can be strapped on or affixed to a stationary object?

 Fact

People have been using dildos for a long time. The first dildos were made of wood, tar, stone, and other materials capable of being molded into phallic shapes firm enough to be used as penetrative sex toys. It is believed that they originated in Asia and date as far back as the Neolithic Period.

Be creative with your dildo. It can be used for more than just penetration. You can use a dildo to stimulate your vulva and clitoris, perineum or anal opening, or use it to caress other erogenous zones. Stroke yourself all over with your dildo. When using a dildo for penetration, play around with different kinds of movements. Review Chapter 11 for tips and techniques on penetration. You can get a dildo to do just what you want it to do without a lot of effort. Play around and see what feels good!

Vibrators

Vibrators are electric or battery-powered devices that are used to relax, massage, and stimulate your body. Most are specifically intended for use on your genitals or other erogenous zones. There are many different kinds of vibrators, designed with different intentions in mind. Some vibrators are designed specifically for vulva and clitoris stimulation, while others are designed to penetrate the vagina or anus. You can also get vibrating dildos that have a built-in vibrating clitoral attachment. Some vibrators were designed as muscle massagers, but work excellently as sex toys. You can even get remote control vibrators and fingertip vibrators!

Vibrators are great when you want to add the intense sensation of vibration to your sexual play. They also come in handy when you are feeling lazy about stimulating yourself manually. They can be particularly useful for women who have never reached orgasm or who have difficulty reaching orgasm. On the other hand, some women find that they can get over-stimulated by vibrators. They are not everyone's cup of tea.

 Alert

When you first begin using a vibrator, it is important to start out on a low setting. Don't overdo the stimulation on the clitoris. You may even want to place a towel or washcloth between your vulva and the vibrator. To get used to the vibration, start on your inner thighs or other body parts before approaching your vulva and clitoris.

Frequent users of vibrators may get addicted to the intense degree of stimulation they supply. While there is no danger of permanently injuring yourself by using a vibrator, you may want to limit your use in order to avoid this scenario. Make sure vibrator use does not keep you from enjoying other forms of stimulation or other routes to orgasm. If you don't have a problem with that, then there is no reason to limit or avoid using a vibrator on a regular basis.

Anal Toys

If you like anal play, anal toys are a great way to enhance your arousal and orgasms. An anal toy is any object designed specifically to pleasure the sphincter muscles of the anus, as well as the prostate gland in men. They can be used at the anal opening, or reach inside the rectum. Butt plugs, anal beads, and anal probes are popular anal toys, in addition to dildos and vibrators designed for anal use. The materials used for anal toys are as varied as those used for dildos. Very important to note, though, is that anything that you use in your anus should have a base or a handle wide enough to keep it from going all the way inside and potentially getting stuck. This is a real danger.

 Essential

It is particularly crucial to keep your anal toys clean, washing them thoroughly with hot water and antibacterial soap after each use. It is also important to make sure that you never use a toy directly from the anus into the vagina without washing it first.

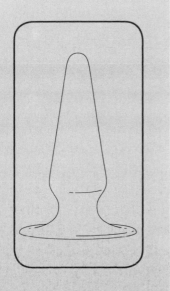

Butt Plugs

Butt plugs are inserted into your anus and simply left there while you continue on with other forms of erotic stimulation. They come in different shapes and sizes, but all should have a flared base to prevent them from getting sucked inside of the rectum. They are typically very narrow just above the base so that the anal sphincter muscle can contract around it and hold it in place inside of you. They then thicken in the middle to ensure a sense of fullness, and narrow at the top to assist in insertion. There are many variations of butt plugs, including vibrating butt plugs, ridged butt plugs, and even inflating butt plugs.

Anal Beads

Anal beads are round, smooth beads strung together on nylon, silicone, or cotton cords. To use them, lubricate each bead and insert them into the anus prior to orgasm. Then pull them out at the time of orgasm. The contractions around each bead as the strand is pulled out can intensify the experience of orgasm. Nylon or silicone cords are best because you can clean them. The cotton cords are for one-time use only.

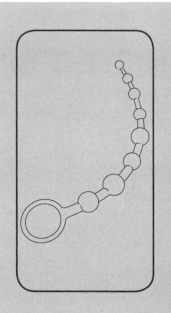

Anal Probes

An anal probe is a device that you use in the anus for a more active experience. They are generally slender, with some kind of ball shape on the insertion end. On the other end they have a handle, enabling you to maneuver the device easily. Move the probe in and out or in any pattern of movement that works for you. There are many variations of anal probes, including vibrating probes and beaded probes, which can function like an anal bead string, when you pull it out at the time of orgasm.

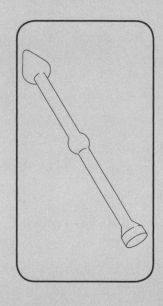

Just for Him

Some toys are made for men, although some of these may greatly benefit female partners as well. Some are designed to enhance a man's pleasure and some are designed to help men provide pleasure to their partners. Not every toy is going to sound or be appealing to every man. Don't get caught in the trap of thinking you need to try or have every device that's ever been made for sexual pleasure. If everything is working great as is, why bother with more stuff? Only choose items that sound appealing to you.

Cock Rings

Cock rings are devices—usually made of leather, metal, or rubber—placed around the base of the penis or around both testicles and the base of the penis, primarily to help maintain a firmer and longer lasting erection. They do this by restricting the blood flow out of the penis. Some men also like them for the unique sensations they help create during arousal and orgasm.

Because you put a cock ring on when you are still soft, there is a little danger that when you become hard, the pressure around the base of your penis will be too much, so it is important to know your girth and get the right size for you, especially if the cock ring you choose is not stretchy or adjustable.

 Alert

> Never leave any cock ring on for more than half an hour because they can cause nerve damage to the penile tissue. Also, you should never use a solid cock ring while using Viagra, because if you cannot go soft, you will not be able to get the cock ring off.

Ball Spreaders

Ball spreaders are a variation of a cock ring that lifts and separates the testicles or stretches the scrotum, providing unique sensations by gently pulling, stretching, and teasing the testicles. These devices are primarily made of leather with metal fasteners. You can also find a version that includes weights to create a heavier pulling sensation on the testicles. Some men find this to be very pleasurable, intensifying their orgasms.

Vagina Simulators

Vagina simulators are devices, either homemade or store bought, which are made to feel like a vagina. They are intended to replicate the sensations of penetration better than just using your hand. There are an infinite number of ways to create your own at home. A plastic baggie filled with lubricant is a simple version of a homemade one. To get some ideas, simply do a web search. You can also purchase vagina simulators that are made of soft material, such as cyber skin. Although they are definitely not the real thing, they come closer than you might imagine. You can even purchase vagina simulators that are built into a life-like mold of a woman's behind.

Penis Pumps

Penis pumps are used to manually pump more blood into the erectile tissue of the penis, helping to create a larger, firmer erection. They work by suction, or siphoning out the air around the penis, and are only intended to help men get and maintain an erection temporarily. They do not have any lasting effects, although some companies like to claim they do. To help maintain your erection using a penis pump, you may also want to use a cock ring, which will keep the blood from flowing out. When choosing a penis pump, it is best to go with a higher end model.

Penis Extensions and Thickeners

You heard it right. Sometimes called penis sleeves, these devices are hollow and attach directly to your penis to either thicken or lengthen it, or assist with intercourse if you have difficulty with erection. They are made from a variety of materials, including cyber skin, latex, and silicone. Some even come with vibrators attached for added pleasure. If you have difficulty maintaining an erection, there are some that can be attached to a strap or a harness to help keep them in place.

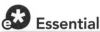 **Essential**

Penis extensions and thickeners are primarily used with the intent of pleasing your lover, which can be emotionally rewarding for you, but may not be as satisfying for you or her in terms of sensation. Be sure your lover is really interested in this before making the investment. She may like your penis just the way it is.

Just For Her

In addition to dildos and vibrators, there are several other sex aids specifically for women. These include clitoral or vaginal pumps, Kegel exercisers, and ben-wa and duo-tone balls. Each of these is designed to help you with your enjoyment of arousal and orgasm.

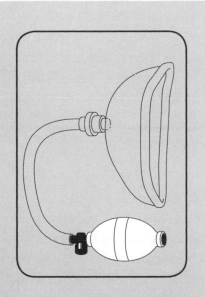

Clitoral or Vaginal Pump

A clitoral or vaginal pump is a device used to manually pump more blood, through suction, into the labia and/or clitoris. It is the female version of the penis pump. It has the potential to increase the intensity of your orgasms. Some come with vibrators, although some women find the combination to be too intense. Be cautious when using these. Follow the directions that come with the product and don't overdo it.

Kegel Exercisers

Kegel exercisers are devices designed specifically to exercise your pelvic floor muscles. In general, you insert them into your vagina and lift, squeeze, and hold before releasing. They come in a variety of forms, made of a variety of materials, including stainless steel and plastic. Some have adjustable resistance, and you can even find some that include a biofeedback device, enabling you to see just how much pressure you are exerting. There are also small vaginal weights that you use to tone your vaginal muscles by gradually increasing the amount of weight you insert.

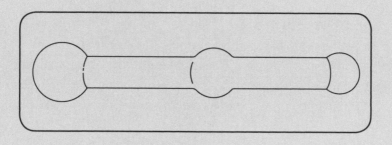

 Fact

Kegel exercisers help increase blood flow to your pelvic area, as well as tone your pelvic floor muscles, which is a sure-fire way to enjoy sex more. While you don't actually need a device to help you exercise your pelvic floor muscles, some women find it helpful, and some of these devices can even double as very effective pleasure tools.

Ben-Wa and Duo-Tone Balls

Ben-wa balls are three-quarter-inch marble-sized balls that you insert into your vagina to increase pleasurable sensations or to exercise your pelvic floor muscles. The original ben-wa balls date back to ancient Japan. Today, there is also a new version called duo-tone balls that are a bit larger—one to one-and-a-half inches—

and attached to each other with a strong nylon cord, which can be tugged on for added pleasure. The cord also aids removal. Duo-tone balls also differ from ben-wa balls in that they are lighter but have a weighted ball bearing inside each ball that helps to create more sensation.

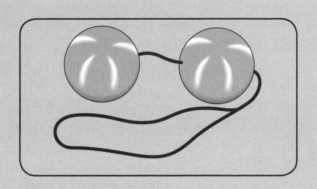

Both ben-wa and duo-tone balls are best used for pleasure when combined with other forms of stimulation, such as a vibrator or vaginal intercourse. Neither should be used anally. If you are using them to strengthen your PC muscle, just insert them and walk around. Your PC muscle will have to work to hold them in place. However, don't wear ben-wa balls out of the house unless you are prepared for a potentially embarrassing situation. Your PC muscle will inevitably grow weary of holding them in place and you may end up losing them while you are out in public. Duo-tone balls would be safer for this because of their size and weight.

Sex Props and Accessories

Sex props and accessories are more peripheral sex aids that are used to assist in a variety of sex acts. These may just add variety and spice to your sex life or they may play a more significant role in helping you reach orgasm.

Sex Props

Sex props are objects that support your body as you engage in sex. There are many commercial props available to assist you in a variety of sexual positions. These include ramps, wedges, cubes, balls, and swings designed specifically for sex. These props can help get you get comfortable in just the right position for your favorite sex act. They may also help you discover some new positions. Of course, if you are on a budget, you can always get creative with your own furniture, pillows, and homemade props.

Textural Delights

If your juices really get flowing through touch, you might like using different textures to stroke or caress your skin. Some options include feathers, fur, wool mitts, leather, latex, and fabrics such as silk, velvet, satin, and chenille. Take turns with your lover lightly stroking or teasing each other. A blindfold can be used to increase the anticipation, which often adds significantly to arousal.

Power Exchange Equipment

Some people have a penchant for power play. Is that you? If so, you are in luck when it comes to props and accessories. Power play equipment can assist you in your role-playing sessions. There are blindfolds and gags to keep your lover from being able to see or talk. Nipple clamps can provide constant nipple stimulation for the women or men who fancy that. Restraints, such as ropes or hand-cuffs, used to keep your lover from using their arms or legs, may be fun to play with. And there are crops, whips, and paddles, used to discipline your lover when he or she has been "naughty." There are many options in this department for those who choose to explore the dark side.

Sex Toy Accessories

As use of sex toys has grown more common, it is no wonder that there are now accessories to go with the most popular toys.

There are harnesses to hold clitoral vibrators in place. There are strap-on harnesses to attach dildos to your body. And there are suction cups to attach a dildo to a surface. In addition, there are miscellaneous attachments that you can add to vibrators to adapt them to different uses.

 Alert

Power exchange should always be mutually consensual. If you are engaging in any kind of power play, it is important to communicate extensively with your lover about safety measures. Because of its darker nature, power play requires extra care and communication in order to build trust and make sure it works for both parties.

Aphrodisiacs

Aphrodisiacs are substances believed to increase sexual desire or libido. Although there is no widely accepted scientific proof of the efficacy of aphrodisiacs, many people claim they have a real effect. Some contain certain nutrients that may support the production of sex hormones in the body. Aphrodisiacs come in the form of food, herbs, spices, drugs, or beverages. Here is a list of substances, by no means comprehensive, that are thought by some to have aphrodisiac properties:

- Almonds
- Asparagus
- Avocado
- Bananas
- Basil
- Cayenne
- Cloves
- Chocolate
- Eggs
- Figs
- Ginseng
- Kava Kava
- Kelp
- Maca
- Mangoes
- Oysters
- Pumpkins
- Tangerines
- Tomatoes
- Vanilla

Some people use drugs, such as marijuana, alcohol, cocaine, amphetamines, and barbiturates, as aphrodisiacs. While these may reduce or altogether eliminate your sexual inhibitions and/or produce pleasurable sensations that cause you to feel sexually aroused, they may actually decrease sexual response and functioning, particularly with moderate-to-heavy use and long-term use. The use or abuse of these substances can also result in more serious harms and/or dependency. You would be wise to stay clear of using any drug as aphrodisiacs.

 Fact

The belief in aphrodisiacs goes way back. The word itself is derived from the name of the Greek goddess of love and beauty, Aphrodite. In folklore, some substances were believed to be aphrodisiacs because of their appearance, namely their resemblance to the male or female genitalia.

The effect of aphrodisiacs may depend on what you believe. The best way to determine whether or not a substance is an aphrodisiac for you is to try it and notice your response. Does the sight, smell, or taste of it turn you on? How do you feel after you partake of it? Scientifically proven or not, if a substance makes you want to have sex, it is deserving of the title *aphrodisiac*, at least on your list. Others will undoubtedly have their own lists.

Music

You may not consider music to be a sex aid, and certainly not all music is capable of inspiring sexual feelings. But some music can, indeed, greatly assist in your arousal and erotic pleasure. Music has the ability to help you get into a flow or a groove that keeps your attention out of your head and into your body.

Different kinds of music work in this way for different people, and at different times. You may like instrumental music without words to help you relax. Or you may want sweet lyrics that connect you to your heart and generate a loving space. You may want something with a strong, rhythmic beat, encouraging you to get your funk on. Or perhaps you like a nice mellow groove that helps you slip into a sensual state of being. Suggestive lyrics or seductive vocals may get you really turned on. Whatever works for you should be duly noted and utilized often to enhance your sexual encounters.

Sexually Explicit Media

Sexually explicit media is the broad umbrella term for any media that depicts explicit or graphic sexual images or descriptions of sexual acts. It includes all adult books, magazines, videos, and websites, both educational and pornographic. It also includes all erotica. There are many ways to use explicit media in helping to build arousal and achieve orgasm, whether you are alone or with a lover. You may use it simply to jumpstart your arousal, or you may use it all the way through to orgasm. You may use it to get new ideas about what to do with your lover, or to learn some new techniques.

Whatever or however you choose to use sexually explicit media is up to you. The use of sexually explicit material is a completely valid sex aid that you should not feel in any way ashamed for using. It is a completely normal activity, and you are certainly not the only one using it.

DIY Explicit Media

Some people like to produce their own sexually explicit media. You may choose photography, videotaping, erotic writing, drawing, or even sculpting. The process of producing your own sexually explicit media with your lover can be very erotic. Afterward, you have a very personalized sex aid for future use when you are alone or even when you are together. Of course, anything you do should be completely consensual, and you should both agree on how the material will be used.

 Alert

Are you concerned that your use of sexually explicit media is excessive or is negatively impacting your life or relationships? If so, consider consulting a therapist. While there is nothing wrong with using erotic images to masturbate or build arousal, compulsive use may cause real problems. Increasing your self-awareness through counseling may help you regain a healthy sense of balance.

Erotica

Erotica refers to literature or art referencing sexuality, usually with the intent to incite sexual desire, while still maintaining a sense of artistry. It is a form of sexually explicit media. It differs from pornography in that it makes a significant artistic statement in addition to being sexy. Erotica generally pays more attention to subtle nuance and details. It often involves some element of fantasy, mystery, or intrigue. The focus of erotica tends to be more on plot, sensuality, character, and relationship development, rather than solely on explicit graphic sexual acts. It is also more likely to include foreplay, intimacy, and mutually satisfying experiences than pornography. Women, in particular, are drawn to erotica for these reasons.

Erotica is often overshadowed in accessibility by pornography, but it is available if you look hard enough. It can come in the form of erotic literature, generally fiction. It may be in one of many sub-genres, such as science fiction, fantasy, horror, or romance. There are also erotic films, both current and dating as far back as the silent film era. There are erotica magazines and journals that include erotic news, reviews, art, photography, fiction, poetry, how-to articles and more. And now, you can even find erotic podcasts and erotic blogs on the Internet.

You may choose to use erotica alone or with a lover. It can be excellent material to fuel your arousal for either self-pleasuring or making love to your partner. Erotica has the potential to open up and stimulate your mind erotically in ways that you may not yet have discovered on your own.

CHAPTER 13

Special Circumstances

Some people are presented with unique challenges when it comes to sex, arousal, and orgasms. There are many special circumstances that can have a significant impact on your sex life. Being challenged with sex in some way, however, does not necessarily mean you cannot enjoy your sexuality. It just means you may need to accept some limitations or work with them. No matter what sexual behaviors you are capable of partaking in, or what sensations your body is capable of experiencing, you can find pleasure, both physical and emotional.

Pregnancy

Being pregnant will undoubtedly affect your sex life, but it does not mean you cannot enjoy your sexuality. In fact, you may enjoy it even more. There are many challenges that couples face with pregnancy, both psychological and physical, but these challenges need not get in the way of your enjoyment of sex; you will just need to adjust yourselves to the new conditions.

One challenge you may face during pregnancy is a fear or concern about you or your baby being hurt in some way. In the past, some doctors believed that women who were pregnant should not have orgasms because they involve uterine contractions and the release of the hormone oxytocin. Both of these could potentially induce labor. We now know, however, that only a small percentage of women need to be concerned about this. Most women can enjoy their orgasms all the way through their pregnancies without any concerns. In fact, some women seek orgasm to help induce labor, and some have even experienced orgasm as a result of labor!

 Fact

During pregnancy, there is increased blood flow into the pelvic region, which can increase the sensation in the genitals and consequently assist in a woman's arousal and enjoyment of orgasm. There have been women who were pre-orgasmic until they got pregnant and many women begin having multiple orgasms during pregnancy.

Your doctor will tell you if you need to be concerned about having orgasms during your pregnancy. Be sure to ask if you are at all worried about it. Under normal conditions, having sex and orgasms while you are pregnant will not hurt you or your baby in any way. In fact, your baby is likely to enjoy the rush of endorphins that are released into your bloodstream upon orgasm.

Another challenge you will face in pregnancy is that of positioning for sex. Pregnant women have limited mobility, and, of course, a protruding abdomen. The missionary position will at some point become uncomfortable. Experiment with new positions. This is the perfect time to explore and engage in female-on-top and rear entry positions.

Once your baby is born, your body will need to heal before you are interested in engaging in most sexual behaviors. The timing is different for every woman. You will also most likely be sleep deprived and very distracted with your newborn infant. Use this time as an opportunity to bond emotionally with your mate; this has the potential to deepen your connection and lovemaking when you get back into it.

Aging

Aging can have a significant impact on your experience of sexuality. Its effects on your sexuality are both psychological and physiological. It is important to adapt to the changes, rather than letting sex drop out of your life. In fact, there are ways in which you could enjoy your sex life even more than when you were younger.

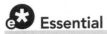 **Essential**

> You do have some control over your enjoyment of sexuality as you age. The more sexually active you are when you are young, the healthier you stay, and the more psychologically adaptable you are to your body's changes, the more likely you are to continue to enjoy your sexuality.

One of the main psychological hurdles you may face is the erroneous belief that older people aren't supposed to be sexual. Many people have the notion that sex is only for young people in their procreative years. Even if you do not hold this belief, you may be worried about what others think. You might feel inhibited by other peoples' expectations that you are no longer sexual.

Another common psychological hurdle is dealing with your body image as your body changes. Influenced by images in the media, you may not think you look sexy or attractive anymore. Aging with a positive attitude, however, can include redefining your concept of attractiveness. You can always find beauty if you look for it in new ways. Remember as well that sex is not really about how you look. The more you can realize that sex is primarily about pleasure and feeling good and that you are entitled to that at any age, the more you will continue to enjoy yourself sexually.

Aging can present many physical hurdles to sex as well, and your overall health has an effect on your ability to have sex. If your back hurts, you tire easily, or you just feel less flexible than you once did, you may not be able to do some of the sexual activities you enjoyed when you were younger. The limitations you feel may have less to do with your genitals than with the rest of your aging body. Keeping your body healthy and well tuned is the only remedy for this.

Aging in Men

As men age, testosterone levels fall. This can affect your sex drive, as well as your experience of getting and maintaining an erection. Unless you have a medical condition, you will still be able to get erections, but they may not be as firm or reliable as they once were. For some men this can be very discouraging. You can cope with these changes in a variety of ways. Some men are proactive, trying everything they can to assist them in arousal and erections. Many find that taking Viagra is often very helpful. Some men give up on sex altogether, deciding that if they can't have it like it once was, it's just not worth having. Other men accept the changes and are willing to work with them. They practice more patience and give themselves the time they need to get aroused and enjoy the erections they are capable of.

Aging brings some benefits to men as well. Older men tend to have more ejaculatory control and can therefore last longer. Another benefit to aging may be an increased enjoyment of emotional intimacy or sensuality, both of which may be more prominent when the need or urge to ejaculate is less strong. If you allow for the possibility that orgasm is not the goal of all sex, as it may have once been for you, you may discover a whole world of pleasures you never realized existed.

Aging in Women

As women get older, they tend to face issues such as vaginal dryness and difficulty with building arousal. Decreased natural lubrication can make intercourse painful. This is easily remedied with the use of personal lubrication, which you may need to rely on more heavily as you age. You may also experience less erotic response to genital and erogenous zone stimulation. Consequently, you may need more stimulation. Vibrators can be particularly helpful. In addition, your pelvic floor muscles are likely to lose their tone as you age. However, if you keep up with your pelvic floor exercises, you can maintain and even improve their tone.

 Fact

> As women age, the depth of the vagina actually decreases, the vaginal walls lose their elasticity, and the labia lose their fullness. These are things that will change how sex feels, but they will not interfere with your ability to get aroused or achieve orgasm.

Some aspects of sex improve for women as they age. Older women have often shed the shame about sex they had when they were young. Thus, they may give themselves more freedom to enjoy their bodies. You may feel more comfortable in your own skin, accept who you are more fully, and no longer need to prove yourself. This can greatly contribute to your ability to surrender to erotic pleasure without any worries of how you will be perceived. Regardless of your age, as long as you still have an interest and desire for sex, you should still be able to find your way to arousal and orgasm.

A New Model for Sex and Aging

Sex is something you can enjoy your whole life. Erotic and sensual pleasure, as well as physical and emotional intimacy, are always available in some way. You may not have the same strength or agility you once had, or the same intensity of sexual responsiveness; but you still have a body capable of giving and receiving immense pleasure, a heart capable of giving and receiving love, and a mind capable of contributing to the arousal of both you and your lover.

To get the most out of it, you may need to take more time with sex as you age. You may even find that your sensual and sexual needs can be met without intercourse. Some couples find that as they age, fondling, caressing, and kissing are perfectly satisfying. You should follow your heart's and your body's impulses and let your sexual encounters be primarily about pleasure and intimacy, not about any specific sexual behavior or sensation. Also, keep in mind that your increasing years give you time to deepen your intimacy, improve your lovemaking skills, and increase your ability to receive and experience more pleasure.

Hormone Replacement Therapy

Hormone replacement therapy is used to either alleviate the effects of hormone depletion or deficiency, or to introduce the hormones of the opposite sex. The use of synthetic hormones is medically controversial and has not been around long enough to determine all of the risks and potential side effects. There are several groups of people that may seek hormone replacement for a variety of reasons. Menopausal women may take estrogen to find relief from menopausal symptoms. Middle-aged men and women may take androgens to counter the effects of aging. Transsexual people may take the hormones of the opposite biological gender, seeking a hormonal experience and/or certain physical attributes more congruent with their gender identity. Intersex people, or people who have mixed gender traits, may elect to take the hormones of one particular gender to enhance those traits in themselves.

Taking synthetic hormones may have a significant effect on your sexuality, influencing libido, arousal, and orgasm. There has not been a tremendous amount of research in this area, but some trends have been identified. Estrogen replacement therapy in menopausal women can assist in vaginal elasticity and lubrication, potentially affecting the quality of arousal and vaginal intercourse. Synthetic estrogen in a transsexual male-to-female can lower libido and tends to change the quality of arousal and orgasm. Men and women taking testosterone for whatever reason are likely to experience an increase in libido and potentially a change in the quality of arousal and orgasm.

 Alert

If you elect to take hormones to enhance your sexuality, there is no guarantee they will have the particular effect you may be seeking. You should always consult a doctor before introducing synthetic hormones into your system, and you will want to weigh the potential benefits with the potential side effects.

Disability, Illness, and Medical Conditions

Having a disability, illness, or medical condition can greatly impact your sex life, but you need not buy into the myth that you cannot still find pleasure and enjoyment in sex. No matter what your circumstances, if you have some interest in being sexual, there is something you can do about it and some erotic or sensual pleasure available to you. Many different diseases, injuries, surgeries, and drugs can potentially interfere with and impair your sexual responsiveness and your ability or desire to engage in various sexual activities.

Effects on Sexuality

There are three distinct ways in which a disability, illness, or medical condition may present challenges to your sex life. First, it could directly affect your reproductive physiology, altering how your sexual organs function. Second, it could affect your general physical ability, making it difficult to engage in or enjoy particular sexual behaviors. And third, your illness or disability may affect you psychologically. It may result in emotional or interpersonal blocks that prevent you from freely enjoying your sexuality.

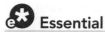 **Essential**

If you have a physical condition that you suspect is affecting your sexuality or if you suspect a medical condition is causing you to experience difficulties with sex, check with your doctor right away. The sooner you know what is going on, the sooner you can tackle the problem.

There are many ways that a disability or medical condition could impair your sexual response. You may experience less desire or arousal. You may lose your ability to ejaculate or orgasm. As a man, you may have erectile difficulty or lack of ejaculatory control. As a woman, you may have increased vaginal dryness. There can also be changes in genital sensation, which could include pain or discomfort, numbness, or burning. This can be unsettling and make you want to avoid focusing any attention whatsoever on your genitals.

A host of general physical health issues that impact your ability to have sex can be present with a disability or illness. General fatigue can rob you of your energy for anything, let alone sexuality. You may have issues with muscle tightness, weakness, spasms, or challenges with mobility or coordination that make it difficult to physically function in particular sexual acts or behaviors. Bladder or bowel dysfunction could present very real challenges to engaging in sex. Numbness, pain, or discomfort anywhere in the body could be so pervasive that it would be hard to direct your attention to enjoying pleasure. Finally, cognitive difficulties can make focusing on sexual pleasure or engaging in a sexual activity a daunting task.

Psychological and emotional challenges may also accompany disability or medical conditions. You may have to deal with society's reaction to your particular disability, circumstance, or predicament.

You may experience self-image or body image issues based on how you perceive yourself or how others perceive you. You may feel less sexy or attractive, less feminine or masculine. You may be less confident about your sexuality or fear being rejected because of your circumstances. You may feel inadequate. You may experience more difficulty communicating with your partner or worry about being able to satisfy her. You may experience mood shifts, depression, anger, or a fear of abandonment or isolation as a result of your condition. You may be feeling guilty about being dependent. Any of these can take their toll on and erode your sex life.

Keys to Enjoying Your Sex Life

There are several keys to enjoying your sex life when you have a disability, illness, or medical condition. The first is to overcome any negative self-perception or feeling that you have about yourself. This process may take time, as self-image issues can be deeply rooted. You may want to consider counseling to support you in this process.

The second key is to adjust your expectations of what sex should look and feel like. You may no longer be able to engage in intercourse. You may have completely lost genital sensation, or be experiencing any number of other limitations or changes. Regardless of your unique circumstances, the more you are able to accept and flow with them, the more likely you will be open to and capable of finding pleasure.

> **EXERCISE:** Use a sensate focus exercise to explore your body in its current state. Spend a couple of hours, alone or with a supportive lover, just exploring different sensations and arousal patterns all over your body. Use different textures and kinds of stimulation. Communicate with your lover about what works for you and what doesn't.

The third key to continuing to enjoy sex is to be open to discovering new paths to erotic or sensual pleasure. You may be limited in the kinds of sexual activities you can engage in or even the kinds of sensations you can feel in your body, but there are many other pleasurable activities and sensations waiting to be discovered. Through your own sexual exploration and discovery, you get to redefine what sex is for you.

The fourth key is to improve your communication skills about both giving and receiving pleasure. This is the perfect opportunity to work on being a better lover. If you put enough attention on it, you could actually improve your skills as a lover and be capable of giving and receiving greater pleasure than ever before.

Pre-Orgasmic Women

Not all women find their path to orgasm easily. There are many reasons for this, both psychological and physiological. If you are not sure if you have ever had an orgasm, then you probably have not. An orgasm is a distinct physiological occurrence that would be hard to miss. While you do not have to orgasm in order to enjoy sex, many women feel as though they are missing out on something. You may start to feel cheated if you don't have the same kind of intense sensations your lover experiences from orgasm.

 Fact

> The Hitachi Magic Wand is a personal massager/vibrator that is often recommended to pre-orgasmic women. The powerful vibrations provide more intense stimulation than you are likely to get with a hand. If you are having difficulty achieving orgasm, you may try this or another vibrator to assist you.

If you are a woman who has never had an orgasm, keep trying. It can take many hours and many attempts over a period of many months to get there, but you will! If you want to orgasm badly enough, it will happen for you. There are many paths. All it takes is some time, some patience, some know-how, and lots of persistence.

The main key to becoming orgasmic is setting aside regular time to pleasure yourself. Give yourself at least two hours, preferably three, to luxuriate in all of the pleasurable sensations you can create in your body. Use your mind, sexual aids, and self-touch. Try masturbating after exercise, when your testosterone levels are up and your body is flooded with endorphins. Start by taking a hot shower or bath to help you relax. If you have already put in a good number of hours trying to bring yourself to orgasm with your own hand to no avail, try using a vibrator.

Low Libido

Some people have very little or no sex drive, or libido. This tends to affect more women than men. It can be caused by numerous factors, both physiological and psychological. For some people, having a low sex drive is not a problem; they are perfectly content with a low libido. Others, however, are troubled by it. They miss having the drive for sex and all of the wonderful feelings and sensations that come with it.

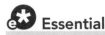 **Essential**

Sometimes the problem with a having a low libido is the discrepancy with your partner's sexual desires and appetite. When this happens you may feel pressured to increase your libido. You will likely be more successful at increasing your libido if you tap into your desire to increase it for your own benefit.

Contributing Factors to Low Libido

Physiological factors for low libido include pain with sex, certain disabilities and medical conditions, and possibly hormonal imbalances. If you suspect any of these to be the cause of your low libido, you should address this first with your physician. If you have ruled out any physiological causes of your low libido, then the issue may be psychological.

Psychological factors for low libido are numerous. Guilt or shame about your sexuality can be strong enough to shut down your sex drive altogether. For some, it may be far easier to repress all sexual feelings than to have ongoing guilt or shame. A history of physical or sexual abuse can also affect libido. Painful memories can make physical intimacy feel unsafe and thus undesirable. Ongoing dissatisfaction with your sexual encounters or difficulty reaching orgasm is likely to decrease your interest in sex. Getting stuck in a rut or becoming bored with your partner can take its toll. Relationship problems also have the ability to negatively impact your sex drive.

Overcoming Low Libido

There is certainly a lot you can do if you want to increase your libido. Tapping into your desire for an increased libido is the first step. Let yourself want to feel more sexual desire. The desire has to stem from inside of you, and it can't be about what you should do or what your lover wants you to do. Finding your own motivation has the potential to open up the gates of arousal.

There is some real wisdom in the phrase "use it or lose it." Libido can be jump-started by engaging more regularly in erotic behavior even when you're not really in the mood. Begin to self-pleasure, even if you don't feel like it. Do your pelvic floor exercises. Seek out sex aids that you sense have the potential to arouse you. Because one of the causes of a low libido is a history of unsatisfying sexual encounters, only engage in sexual encounters that you will enjoy. If you have a history of physical or sexual abuse, you should consider seeking some professional counseling to help you unravel the negative impact it is having on your sexuality.

Pain with Sex

Both men and women can suffer from pain with sex, particularly intercourse. Such pain is more common in women. There are many different kinds of pain and many potential causes. Needless to say, pain with sex will inevitably affect the quality of your sexual interactions. It can interfere with arousal and orgasm, and it will likely affect your libido in the long run.

 Alert

If you experience pain with sex, you should seek medical attention from a gynecologist or urologist, preferably one that specializes in pelvic pain. If a doctor tells you there is nothing wrong with you but you still experience pain, find another doctor who can help you.

If you or your lover is experiencing pain with sex, it is important to stop any sexual behavior that is causing the pain. Continuing a sexual behavior when it is painful can cause you to become disinterested in that particular behavior and perhaps other sexual behaviors as well. Painful sex can also have a negative impact on your relationship. Only engage in sexual behaviors that feel good to both of you and seek medical attention to deal with any physical problems.

Lack of Ejaculatory Control

Early ejaculation, premature ejaculation, and rapid ejaculation all describe the problem of not having the amount of control you desire over your ejaculation. You may want to be able to delay ejaculation so that you can prolong intercourse or other sex play that requires an erection. It can be frustrating not to have control of the timing of your ejaculation.

Early ejaculation affects a lot of men at some point or other in their lives. It is very common in young men who are just beginning to explore their sexuality. It can also happen with men of any age, particularly if you have not had much sex recently, if you have performance anxiety, or if you are in some way challenged by your relationship dynamics. Fortunately, lack of ejaculatory control is rarely the result of a physiological problem.

Ways to Improve Ejaculatory Control

Ejaculation control is a skill that can be learned. Mastery over your ejaculation is best gained by experimenting while self-pleasuring. Start by masturbating until you are close to orgasm. Carefully notice the sensations that tell you your orgasm is approaching. When you can identify these sensations, you know when you need to distract yourself or stop the stimulation if you want to delay orgasm. After you have mastered deciding when and when not to orgasm during masturbation, you can begin experimenting with a partner. The challenge then is to assert yourself in whatever way you need to control the stimulation you are receiving.

 Fact

Being able to recognize the point of no return or ejaculatory inevitability is the primary key to learning ejaculatory control. When you understand your body's sexual response from the inside, you can learn to master it, using such techniques as self-distraction and the stop-and-start technique.

There are two simple ways to decrease your arousal when you feel orgasm may be approaching, self-distraction and the stop-and-start technique. In self-distraction, you mentally distract yourself from the pleasurable sensations. You can think of things that have a neutralizing effect on your arousal, keeping it in a holding pattern, or that actually have a counter-effect and decrease your arousal. This works to delay ejaculation for some. The stop-and-start technique involves stopping any genital stimulation before you reach the point of ejaculatory inevitability, taking a break and resuming stimulation until you approach that point again.

Other methods include the squeeze technique, wherein you squeeze the penis hard just below the glans for twenty to thirty seconds just before you feel you are about to come. Do this several times before you finally let yourself ejaculate. Doing pelvic floor exercises can also help significantly with ejaculatory control. If your PC muscle gets strong enough, you should be able to control ejaculation by simply squeezing it just before the point of no return. Yet another method is to desensitize your penis with the use of thicker condoms, two condoms, or desensitizing cream. The creams will also affect your lover, so make sure she is okay with that.

Erectile Difficulty

Men can have difficulty both getting and maintaining an erection. For many men, erections are a symbol of virility. It can therefore be very upsetting to be deprived of that potent feeling. If you have always had erectile difficulty, you may accept your circumstance more, although it may still be a source of anguish for you. If you only have difficulty occasionally, it may be very hard to adjust to when it happens. Some men have an easier time psychologically dealing with erectile difficulty, regardless of how or when they experience it.

Physiological Solutions

There are many strategies for dealing with erectile difficulty on a physiological level. Some men use medication to help them achieve erection. For many, this is a fairly reliable way to obtain an erection. It comes with some risky and challenging side effects, however, such as headaches, visual impairment, and possible heart attack. Some men use devices such as penis pumps or cock rings. This also can lead to positive results without the same degree of risk as drugs. Some men, however, have an aversion to the use of such devices. They may prefer to deal with the problem psychologically.

Psychological Causes and Solutions

Erectile difficulty is sometimes the result of a medical condition or aging, but the problem can also be psychological or interpersonal. Knowing the cause will help in assessing what kind of treatment may help. To figure this out, ask yourself whether the erectile difficulty happens primarily with a lover or if it also occurs during self-pleasuring. If everything works fine when you are self-pleasuring, then chances are the cause is emotional or interpersonal.

Interpersonal difficulties are common. Men often don't realize when their preconditions for having sex are not met. Most people need to feel comfortable with their partner for their bodies to perform naturally. Your mind might say yes to sex, but your body may not be ready if you do not feel emotionally safe. Lack of erection can be a sign that your mind and your emotions are in conflict. If you are having difficulties in your relationship, particularly with intimacy, you may want to see a couples' counselor who specializes in sexuality.

 Essential

Whatever your particular circumstance and whatever route you choose to deal with your erectile difficulty, it is especially important to be gentle with yourself and to keep an open mind. Be willing to seek professional help, try different treatments or strategies, and explore your feelings more deeply.

If the erectile difficulty occurs while self-pleasuring, there still could be an emotional cause. You may be unconsciously carrying around some shame about sex or you may have fears of being an inadequate lover. Unfortunately, erectile inconsistency can itself lead to performance anxiety. This anxiety can make getting an erection even more difficult. If you are experiencing this kind of negative spiral, it is important to get support. Stop and talk with your partner about how you feel and what you need. When you become more skilled at meeting your preconditions for sex, your sexual functioning is bound to go more smoothly.

CHAPTER 14

Enhancing Your Orgasms

T here are orgasms and then there are *orgasms*. Many people are perfectly satisfied with their ordinary run-of-the-mill orgasms. They don't feel the need to ask if there could be something even more intense. Some erotic pioneers, however, have discovered erotic states of arousal that go beyond the kinds of experiences most people normally have with sex and orgasm. These new possibilities are yours to dive into and explore if you wish.

Multiple Orgasms

There is no reason why anyone should settle for just one orgasm when both men and women are capable of experiencing numerous orgasms within a single sexual encounter. Sometimes one good orgasm is all you need, but when there is more in you that wants to be released, then why not go for it?

Multiple orgasm is the experience of having two or more orgasms in succession without leaving the arousal phase. The intensity, number, duration, and distance between each orgasm can vary widely. To understand what multiple orgasms are, it is important to remember that one orgasm consists of many contractions. Do not confuse each contraction for an orgasm. There is a difference between having a long orgasm and having multiple orgasms. In multiple orgasms there is some buildup for each successive orgasm, much like the build up for your first orgasm, although it may take considerably less time.

Multiple orgasms are more common for women. Men, however, are also capable of experiencing successive orgasms. Becoming multi-orgasmic is simply a matter of practice. If you are determined and follow certain practices, you may be able to find your way there.

Multiple Orgasms for Her

If you are a woman who relies on clitoral stimulation for orgasm, as most women do, let your clitoris rest as long as it needs to after your first orgasm. You can stimulate other parts of your body, or continue to engage in penetration for a while before going for your next orgasm. If your clitoris remains too sensitive, then you may need to back off of clitoral stimulation altogether and work on increasing your arousal in other ways. Once your clitoris will tolerate more stimulation, you can start in again. If you can pick up the thread of arousal you may find your way to orgasm again in a matter of minutes. But take your time; the more time you spend increasing your arousal, the more intense your orgasm is likely to be. Don't try to force it. This is just about your pleasure, what feels good to you.

Multiple Orgasms for Him

If you are a man, being able to experience multiple orgasms requires that you learn to refrain from ejaculation. Essentially, you must separate your orgasm from your ejaculation. In order to do this you will need to intimately understand your body's sexual response and gain control over ejaculatory inevitability, or the point of no return. By strengthening your PC muscle and squeezing it really hard at the onset of orgasm, you can stop yourself from ejaculating while still allowing yourself to orgasm. Ejaculation is what initiates the refractory period. Thus, if you bypass ejaculation, you can maintain your erection and be able to continue having orgasms. This process can repeat until you are ready to allow yourself to ejaculate. It takes a lot of self-discipline, but many men and their lovers have found it to be a very worthwhile practice.

G-Spot Orgasm and Female Ejaculation

More and more women are discovering the intense pleasures of the G-spot orgasm and female ejaculation. Some women find their way to these experiences by accident, simply the result of enjoying sex and doing what feels good. Other women hear about such experiences and then seek to create them for themselves, following the suggestions of the women who have gone there before. Many women who have experienced G-spot orgasm and female ejaculation proclaim that they are deeply satisfying and make for more enjoyable orgasms. This is often enough to make other women want to get in on the action.

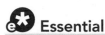 **Essential**

> Many women find that they need to simultaneously stimulate their clitoris in order to achieve G-spot orgasm. This may actually result in a blended orgasm—double bonus! The sensations experienced from a G-spot orgasm are notably different from clitoral orgasms; they feel much fuller and deeper.

G Marks the Spot

A G-spot orgasm refers to an orgasm that results from the stimulation of the sensitive tissue of the G-spot, the area on the front wall of the vagina about one to two inches inside the vaginal canal. It is possible to stimulate the G-spot from the outside as well by putting pressure directly above the pubic mound. The G-spot is most likely to respond to stimulation once you are already significantly aroused. If you try stimulating it before you are turned on, it may feel sensitive in a way that is irritating. When stimulating the G-spot from inside the vaginal canal, making a come-hither motion with one or two fingers inserted should do the trick. You may also want to explore other kinds of stimulation to the G-spot, including vaginal penetration with a penis or sex toy.

Letting Your Waters Flow

Female ejaculation is the sudden release of fluids from the urethra during orgasm. Often it results from G-spot stimulation. The fluids released in female ejaculation are not urine. Laboratory analysis has shown that female ejaculate may have some of the same components as urine, but there is a significant difference in the composition.

The amount of ejaculate released and the way in which it is expelled from the urethra can vary tremendously. It can be as little as two drops or as much as two cups. The fluid may dribble out, gush out, or squirt and spray. Female ejaculation may occur with or without G-spot stimulation, but it usually requires a high state of arousal.

Certain foundational practices can assist you in your ability to ejaculate. Do your pelvic floor exercises to strengthen your PC muscle. You can also learn to play with erotic energy in your body, circulating it rather than expelling it. Learn to let it increase and build to greater and greater heights. Another foundational practice is to work on deepening intimacy and improving communication with your lover. Each of these things will support you in letting your waters flow.

 Fact

The fluid that is released during female ejaculation is believed to originate from the Skene's or paraurethral glands at the base of the urethra, near the front wall of the vagina and/or the bladder. Since all women have paraurethral glands, it is believed that all women produce ejaculate, whether or not they expel it from their body during orgasm.

Once you have done some of the foundational work, you can begin to play with the actual strategies for ejaculating. To prepare, lay down plenty of towels so you won't worry about making a mess. Make sure your bladder is empty before you attempt to ejaculate so you don't worry that you are just going to pee. Spend lots of time building arousal doing whatever activities get you the most turned on. Once you are really turned on, and your vagina and vulva are significantly engorged with blood, you or your lover can begin to stimulate your G-spot, either with fingers or a sex toy. When the G-spot is fully aroused and swollen, it will put pressure on the urethra and make you feel like you have to pee. This is your cue to relax into the sensation until you flood yourself with your own nectar. Once you have accomplished this gushing technique, you can practice pushing your PC muscle out, directing the fluid to squirt.

Can Every Woman Have These Experiences?

Some sex experts believe any woman can learn to ejaculate and some are doubtful. Many women have no interest in trying. Of those who try, not all are successful. The only way to know if you are capable of or would enjoy ejaculating is trying it. You can follow the practices mentioned here to help guide you. It will probably take some practice. Be sure to focus on increasing or expanding your pleasure. If you can accomplish that, you are doing great, whether or not you ejaculate.

Power Exchange

A very powerful, highly erotic, and often feared sexual practice is that of power exchange, sometimes referred to as power play. Power exchange is a mutually consensual type of sexual role-play, wherein one partner has control or power over the other partner. There are many names and variations for this kind of play, including topping and bottoming, bondage and discipline, dominant and submissive, master and slave, and sadism and masochism. Power exchange may involve restriction of movement, sensory depriva-tion, psychological dominance, or inflicting strong sensation or pain. It may or it may not include any actual direct genital stimula-tion. Power exchange is sometimes acted out in what is known as a "scene," a role-play scenario that is plotted out ahead of time, with all parties agreeing to the terms and conditions.

 Alert

> You should only engage in power exchange if you choose it yourself and you are doing it with someone you trust. Never let yourself get pressured or coaxed into any sexual behavior. Keep your communica-tion channels open and share what is working and what is not. Make sure you feel listened to and respected.

Surrendering to a power exchange is not for everyone. Most peo-ple like to feel like they have control of their own experience. They are reluctant to trust someone else to take charge, especially when it comes to such a vulnerable act as sex. However, for some, letting another take responsibility for their arousal is an extreme turn-on. It essentially allows them to do nothing but surrender to the experi-ence and the sensations that come their way. People who engage in this kind of sex play often find that the arousal they build up during a scene can make for very powerful orgasms. Some scenes go on for quite some time, allowing for the arousal to build to very high states.

Power exchange can be very intense. The degree of trust and surrender that goes into giving your lover complete control can generate a tremendous feeling of vulnerability. Such strong feelings can heighten the sense of connection between the two of you. The person who has control often feels very powerful, having gained his lover's trust. But he may feel vulnerable too, because of his desire to perform well for his lover. The person who surrenders control often feels vulnerable because he is, to some degree, at the mercy of his lover. He may also feel powerful because he is brave enough to hand over control. Because of these dynamics, people engaging in power exchange often report very emotional experiences with orgasm.

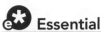 **Essential**

Everyone has access to both masculine and feminine traits and qualities. You may put a great value on balancing these energies within
yourself and in your daily life. Regardless of how you are in the rest of
your life, you may choose to gravitate to one pole or the other in your
sexuality. This is completely acceptable.

The Fine Art of Polarity

A more tempered version of power exchange is evident when couples play with the polarity of masculine and feminine energy. One lover may embody the masculine archetype and the other may embody the feminine archetype. This polarity can make for very hot chemistry. Playing with gender polarity is something many people do quite naturally, without even thinking about it. It is possible, how-ever, to cultivate it as a conscious practice. It starts with acknowledg-ing your core essence (masculine or feminine), embracing it, and letting that guide you in your sexuality and your sexual encounters.

The masculine archetype, or the top, takes charge of the sex-ual encounter, guiding it and directing it, whereas the feminine, or the bottom, surrenders, following in the direction that the mascu-line leads. Of course, in order for this to work, the feminine partner needs to trust that the masculine will lead well, attending to her needs in an effort to satisfy her. Likewise, the masculine partner needs to trust that he will be granted that control and appreciated in his role. When both lovers are able to embody their masculine and feminine roles during sex, magic can happen.

Playing with Power

Power exchange can be as scary as it is exciting. You may want to get your feet wet first to see if you like it. Play with the roles briefly by using a blindfold. One of you will take control as the giver, while the other will surrender control as the receiver. With the receiver blindfolded, the giver can apply light touch and caressing at first. The receiver can focus on surrendering, relaxing, and receiving pleasure. As the giver, focus on your lover's responsiveness to your touch. Notice what seems to be working and what doesn't.

The giver should ask for feedback from time to time. As the receiver, see if you can wait to give feedback until you are asked. The only exception is if you are being tremendously annoyed by some aspect of the experience. Part of surrendering control is releasing your expectations and being able to enjoy whatever your lover is offering you in that moment. If you are feeling adventuresome and would like to try more types of sensation, you can add other kinds of erotic touch: pinching, spanking, or slapping. Go at your own pace and only explore in a way that will not harm your relationship in any way.

Expansive Orgasmic Experiences

If you've ever thought that there could be more to sex, then you are probably right. An expansive orgasm is an experience that makes you feel like you are finally approaching your full potential for orgasmic bliss. They are within reach, but you will need to do some groundwork in order to open those channels within you.

Expansive orgasmic experiences go beyond what would be considered a regular genital orgasm. Typical genital orgasms last approximately 3–5 seconds in men and 5–10 seconds in women. They are marked by a series of strong pelvic contractions and a sense of release or "going over the edge." The focus of pleasurable sensations is primarily in the pelvis and genitals. An expansive orgasm is longer in duration and may include a variety of pleasurable sensations felt throughout the body. It may or may not include the same sense of release. Because of its extended duration, the experience is more like a state than an event. There are many different variations of expansive orgasm. Some of the most common names for these experiences are expanded orgasms, full body orgasms, extended massive orgasms, energy orgasms, transcendent orgasms, and Tantric orgasms.

 Essential

> Expansive orgasms are indeed their own brand of orgasm. In fact, they are distinct enough from what most of us think of as orgasms that they deserve a separate category altogether. The physiological response of expansive orgasms can be quite different but can only be described in subjective terms.

Just as there are many different ways one might experience a genital orgasm, there are many ways to experience expansive orgasms. Some may feel more energetic, with minimal genital sensation or involvement. The experience is like waves of energy coursing through your entire being, causing your spine to undulate. These waves give you a sense of energetic release and freedom.

Other types of expanded orgasm may have a tremendous amount of erotic charge built into them, spreading warmth and electricity from your genitals outward in all directions. They give you the sense that your entire being is charged with ecstatic energy. They can be understood as a heightened state of arousal that can last for an extended period of time.

Finally, some expanded orgasms combine a genital orgasm with an energetic kind of orgasm. Your entire body experiences the intensity of the orgasmic release as it moves in waves up and down your spine, spreading its warmth and ecstatic vibration throughout your entire being.

Many people experience expansive orgasms as more emotional or spiritual than typical genital orgasms. They are often accompanied with a sense of timelessness. They may include a profound sense of connection or oneness with your lover, your surroundings, and all of life. Some people happen upon such states from their own exploration. Others seek them out and get there by following specific practices.

Preparations for Expansive Orgasmic Experiences

There are some preparations that can assist you in finding your way to the various types of expanded orgasm. These preparations may take time to master. They involve opening the body in ways that might be new to you. Practice is necessary in order to develop your capacity for expanded orgasm.

Opening Your Mind

The first way to prepare is to open your mind to the possibility of greater and more intense pleasure. If your mind is not open, you will most likely continue the same patterns and routines with sex that you always have. Consequently, you will keep having the same kinds of experiences.

 Alert

When working with your breath, strong emotions can emerge. Be prepared for any number of feelings and sensations that may arise from simply breathing more deeply. You may find that your body begins to quiver and shake, or you may be flooded with tears or laughter. This is all par for the course and part of releasing energy blocks.

Breath Awareness and Expansion

The second preparation is to bring more awareness to your breath. By focusing on your breath and allowing it to deepen, you will come more into your body and the sensations there. This will also help you access more profoundly relaxed states. You will also become more aware of energy flowing within your body. With this awareness you can begin to release blocks to the flow of this energy. The more conscious you can be of your breath, the more you can use it in a way to assist you in building arousal and expanding the orgasmic energy when the time comes.

Circulating or Streaming Energy

The third preparation is learning to circulate or stream energy through your body. Once you are open and aware of energy in your body, you can begin to consciously amplify it. By channeling and recirculating energy, you can allow it to build until you feel fully charged. This will enable you to experience energy coursing through your entire being. You may experience the energy starting at the base of the spine, traveling all the way up the spine. It may then shoot out the top of your head. Alternatively, the energy may recycle by traveling back down the front of your body to create a continuous loop.

The Journey to Expansive Orgasm

Once you have done some preparation and feel energetically open, you can begin to set a greater intention to experience more expansive orgasms. The following practices can help open the channels within you to such states. These practices can be done alone or with a partner. You should set aside at least two hours, if not three or four. You will be making love to yourself or your lover, and all of the sexual behaviors that you normally engage in can be a part of this practice. It is less about the particular activities and more about the energy you allow to flow within you. You don't have to engage in all of these practices in one encounter. In fact, in the beginning it is probably best to pick just one as your primary focus. You can gradually integrate all three.

Containing More Arousal

Having expansive orgasms requires that you contain high states of arousal. Your ability to deepen your breath and circulate your energy will help tremendously with this, as will your ability to simply relax into pleasurable sensations. You want to be able to stay present with and keep inviting in more sensation. If it feels like too much at any point, go back to focusing on your breathing. In comparison, when you go for a genital orgasm, you are looking to climax and then dissipate your energy. Instead, expanded orgasm practices seek to sustain a high state of energy and arousal, without looking to discharge it.

Spreading the Sweet Spot

As you focus on the pleasurable sensations in your genitals, you can begin to allow that pleasure to spread to the tissues nearby. This can be aided by varying the stimulation to make it lighter and broader. It also helps to focus on relaxing the tissues in the rest of your body, inviting all areas to open and receive the pleasure. See how far you can spread the ecstatic sensations into the rest of your being.

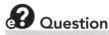 **Question**

Can I experience expansive orgasms all by myself?
Yes, you can. You don't need a lover to help you access expansive orgasmic states. But you do need to devote a fair amount of time to indulging yourself in pleasure. A partner can help you keep building your arousal, but your own touch and imagination may be quite sufficient.

Expand Your Sense of Connection and Oneness

Expanding a sense of connection and oneness to your lover, your surroundings, and all of life will support a more expansive orgasmic experience. If you are with a lover, you can practice being present with each other by looking into each other's eyes and breathing together. See if you can feel each other's energy bodies. Let yourselves feel your desire for each other. Let it fill you. Breathe it in. Sometimes this is all it takes to help you access more expansive states.

APPENDIX A

Glossary

Anal Intercourse A sexual act in which a man inserts his penis into another person's anus.

Anal Play Any anal stimulation or penetration using a penis, fingers, tongue, or sex toy.

Analingus A method of anal or oral sex, also known as anal-oral contact, in which one person's mouth and tongue are used to stimulate another person's anus.

Aphrodisiac A substance believed to increase sexual desire; it can be from a physical or emotional source.

BDSM An abbreviation for Bondage and Discipline and Sadism and Masochism, forms of power exchange.

Cunnilingus Oral stimulation of the female genitals.

Erogenous Zone Areas of the body with heightened sensitivity; stimulation of these areas results in arousal and/or sexual response.

Erotica Literature or art referencing sexuality, usually with the intent to incite sexual desire, while still maintaining a sense of artistic endeavor.

Estrogen The predominant female hormone.

Explicit Media Any media that depicts explicit or graphic sexual images or descriptions of sexual acts.

Fellatio Oral stimulation of the male genitals.

Fingering Using one's fingers to stimulate the clitoris, vagina, or anus.

Foreplay Any erotic stimulation between lovers that comes before sexual intercourse.

Genitals External sex organs.

G-Spot A sexually sensitive area on the upper wall of the vagina approximately two inches from the vaginal opening that when stimulated can lead to orgasm and female ejaculation.

Hand Job Manual stimulation; the use of a hand to stimulate the penis or the vulva.

Intercourse A sexual act in which the penis is inserted into the vagina or anus.

Kegels Exercises to strengthen the pelvic floor muscles.

Libido Sexual desire or sex drive.

Masturbation Sexually pleasing one's genitals through self-stimulation.

Menopause The process of the termination of a woman's menstrual cycle and reproductive capacity.

Multiple Orgasm Having several orgasms occurring in succession.

Orgasm Sexual climax with intense pleasure, usually accompanied by a series of involuntary contractions of the sexual organs, the anus, and the pelvic muscles.

Pegging A sexual act in which a female penetrates a man's anus with a strap-on dildo.

Personal Lubricant A synthetic slippery substance applied to the genitals, erogenous zones, or fingers to assist in stimulation and penetration.

Power Exchange A mutually consensual type of sexual role-play, wherein one partner has control or power over the other partner.

Pre-Orgasmic Not having yet experienced orgasm.

P-Spot A sexually sensitive part of the prostate gland in the lower rectum of men; Similar to the female G-spot

Self-Pleasuring Erotic solo play; masturbation.

Sex Aid Any item used to help increase sexual desire or enhance sexual pleasure, such as explicit media, sex toys, or props.

Sex Toy Object used to enhance pleasure during sexual acts, such as a dildo, cock ring, or vibrator.

STD/STI Sexually transmitted disease/Sexually transmitted infections; diseases or infections that have been transmitted through sexual contact.

Tantra A form of yoga based on Hindu or Buddhist philosophy whose goal is to achieve ecstasy or nirvana through esoteric and sometimes erotic practices; sexual union of a woman and man; Sanskrit for *woven together.*

Testosterone The predominant male sex hormone, also found in smaller quantities in women.

Vasocongestion The accumulation of blood in the genital tissues as a result of sexual excitement, causing swelling and erection. Also referred to as *engorgement.*

Additional Resources

Internet Resources

www.eartherotics.com
An online boutique offering eco-logically friendly sex toys and accessories.

www.goodvibes.com
Good Vibrations offers a plethora of toys, movies, gifts and gift cards, various body products, books, and more; it features an online magazine, articles, and blogs, and offers various links including a link to on-demand videos.

www.hai.org
Human Awareness Institute (HAI) is located in several regions around the world. HAI strives to empower individuals as loving, aware, confident, and interdependent beings by providing workshops on love, intimacy, and sexuality.

www.loveyoursexlife.com
Clinical Sexologist Dr. Amy Cooper, PhD, offers coaching for individuals or couples, focusing on issues such as difficulty with orgasm, erectile difficulty, loss of interest in sex, concerns about sexual orientation, and body image issues, as well as developing skills in intimacy and sexual creativity.

www.plannedparenthood.org
Planned Parenthood offers community resources for sexual and reproductive health care for men, women, and teens in all fifty states. They offer comprehensive information online about abortion, birth control, pregnancy, relationships, sex, STDs, and many other topics.

www.scarleteen.com
A sex education website designed specifically for teens. It includes an array of information, such as sexual anatomy, sexual health links, interactive posts, and blogs.

www.sexuality.org
Dedicated to positive sexual expression, this site offers guides and reviews on sex toys, educational and erotic books, and videos; it features a sex *City Guide* set of links to popular U.S. cities, including guides to clubs, adult shops, sex education, and sexuality-spirituality based contacts, as well as LGBT resources, support groups, and events.

www.siecus.org
Sexuality Information and Education Council of the U.S. (SIECUS), a national nonprofit organization, offers comprehensive information on many issues such as teen pregnancy, sexual orientation, and STD prevention, as well as a variety of links to important resources, articles, and news.

www.slinkyproductions.com
Catherine Rose's Slinky Productions: An exotic dance school for women in San Francisco, California, offering classes in lap dancing, pole dancing, floor shows, and exotic dancing techniques; it also features an online store with DVDs, books, and additional resources.

www.tantra.com
This site offers extensive information on Tantra practices, history, yoga, sex, and massage, as well as techniques of the Kama Sutra; it also offers audio and video media, an online store, personals, e-books, articles, and resources for workshops.

www.vitalhealth.com
The Vital Health Institute, run by Dr. Andrew Cook, MD, FACOG, specializes in treating women with pelvic pain and endometriosis. They are a renowned international institute located in Los Gatos, California.

Additional Reading

Anand, Margo. *The Art of Sexual Ecstasy: The Path of Sacred Sexuality for Western Lovers* (Los Angeles, CA: Jeremy P. Tarcher, Inc., 1989).

Blue, Violet. *The Ultimate Guide to Cunnilingus: How to Go Down on a Woman and Give Her Exquisite Pleasure* (San Francisco, CA: Cleis Press, 2002).

Blue, Violet. *The Ultimate Guide to Fellatio: How to Go Down on a Man and Give Him Mind-Blowing Pleasure* (San Francisco, CA: Cleis Press, 2002).

Butler, Robert N. and Myrna I. Lewis, PhD. *The New Love and Sex after 60* (NY: Ballantine Books, 2002).

Dodson, Betty, PhD. *Sex for One: The Joy of Self loving* (New York, NY: Three Rivers Press, 1996).

Ellison, Carol Rinkleib, PhD. *Women's Sexualities: Generations of Women Share Intimate Secrets of Sexual Self-Acceptance* (Oakland, CA: New Harbinger Publications, Inc., 2000).

Heiman, Julia R. and Joseph and Leslie LoPiccolo. *Becoming Orgasmic: A Sexual Growth Program for Women* (Englewood Cliffs, NJ: Prentice-Hall, Inc., 1976).

Henkin, William A. and Sybil Holiday. *Consensual Sadomasochism: How to Talk About It and How to Do It Safely* (Los Angeles, CA: Daedalus Publishing Company, 1996).

Kaufman, Miriam, MD, Fran Odette and Cory Silverberg. *The Ultimate Guide to Sex And Disability: For All of Us Who Live with Disabilities, Chronic Pain and Illness* (San Francisco, CA: Cleis Press, 2007).

Litten, Harold, Dr. *The Joy of Solo Sex* (Mobile, AL: Factor Press, 1993).

Pokras, Somraj and Jeffre Talltrees. *Female Ejaculation: Unleash the Ultimate G-Spot Orgasm.* (Berkeley, CA: Amorata Press, 2009).

Semans, Anne and Cathy Winks. *The Good Vibrations Guide to Sex* (Pittsburg, PA: Cleis Press, Inc., 1994).

Taylor, Patricia, PhD. *Expanded Orgasm: Soar to Ecstasy at Your Lover's Every Touch* (Naperville, IL: Sourcebooks, Inc., 2002).

Index